Mental Illness, Dementia and Family in China

With rapid economic progress and increasing life expectancy in East Asian societies, more attention is being paid by their governments, the media and the academy to mental illness and dementia. While clinical research on mental illness and dementia in Chinese societies acknowledges the importance of culture in shaping people's experiences of these illnesses, how Chinese culture shapes people's understandings of and responses to mental illness and dementia has yet to be interrogated to any depth.

Mental Illness, Dementia and Family in China breaks new ground in exploring how Chinese culture, namely, the understandings, norms, values and scripts that people acquire through being members of a Chinese community, shapes contemporary stories of mental illness, dementia and family caregiving. This book is innovative in examining and comparing stories which have been drawn from both real life ('life stories'), as well as from film and television productions ('filmic stories'). These two forms effectively complement each other, with life stories generally presenting an 'insider's' account and filmic stories generally presenting an 'outsider's' account. What remains unvoiced in one kind of story may be voiced in the other kind. Drawing on the perspectives and analytic approaches of narrative analysis and cultural studies, Guy Ramsay uncovers culturally shaped continuities and departures in representations of time, identity and cause of illness as well as in the language employed in contemporary stories of mental illness, dementia and family caregiving in China.

This book will be invaluable to students and scholars working on Chinese cultural studies and Asian social policy, as well as those interested in psychiatry, mental health and disability studies more broadly.

Guy Ramsay is Senior Lecturer in Chinese Language and Studies at the University of Queensland, Australia.

Routledge/Asian Studies Association of Australia (ASAA) East Asia Series

Edited by Tessa Morris-Suzuki and Morris Low

Editorial Board: Professor Geremie Barmé (Australian National University), Emeritus Professor Colin Mackerras (Griffith University), Professor Vera Mackie (University of Wollongong) and Professor Sonia Ryang (University of Iowa).

This series represents a showcase for the latest cutting-edge research in the field of East Asian studies, from both established scholars and rising academics. It will include studies from every part of the East Asian region (including China, Japan, North and South Korea and Taiwan) as well as comparative studies dealing with more than one country. Topics covered may be contemporary or historical, and relate to any of the humanities or social sciences. The series is an invaluable source of information and challenging perspectives for advanced students and researchers alike.

Routledge is pleased to invite proposals for new books in the series. In the first instance, any interested authors should contact:

Professor Tessa Morris-Suzuki
School of Culture, History and Language
Australian National University
Canberra, ACT0200 Australia

Associate Professor Morris Low
School of Languages and Comparative Cultural Studies
University of Queensland
Brisbane, QLD 4072, Australia

Routledge/Asian Studies Association of Australia (ASAA) East Asia Series

This book is dedicated with much love to Luther King A. Tambaoan.

Mental Illness, Dementia and Family in China

Guy Ramsay

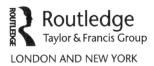
Routledge
Taylor & Francis Group

LONDON AND NEW YORK

First published 2013 by Routledge

2 Park Square, Milton Park, Abingdon, Oxfordshire OX14 4RN
52 Vanderbilt Avenue, New York, NY 10017

Routledge is an imprint of the Taylor & Francis Group, an informa business

First issued in paperback 2019

British Library Cataloguing in Publication Data
A catalogue record for this book is available from the British Library

Library of Congress Cataloging in Publication Data
Ramsay, Guy Malcolm.
Mental illness, dementia and family in China / Guy Ramsay.
pages cm. -- (Routledge/Asian Studies Association of Australia (ASAA)
East Asia series)
Includes bibliographical references and index.
1. Mental health policy--China. 2. Mental health services--China. 3.
Mentally ill--Family relationships--China. I. Title.
RA790.7.C6R36 2013
362.168'30951--dc23
2012037498

ISBN: 978-0-415-81006-7 (hbk)
ISBN: 978-0-367-89901-1 (pbk)

Typeset in Times New Roman
by Saxon Graphics Ltd, Derby

Contents

Acknowledgements

I wish to thank the following people and organisations for their kind assistance in the development and writing of this monograph: Ping Chen, Helen Creese, Jill Halil, Mark Hayward, Joanne Hopper, Daphne Hsieh, Wendy Jiang, Leong Ko, Brenda Liang, Morris Low, Abigail Loxham, Wai Wai Lui, Juliana de Nooy, Veronica Pearson, Judith Ramsay, John Traphagan, Lara Vanderstaay and Carol Wical; and Beijing University Number Six Hospital, Hong Kong Alzheimer's Disease Association, the Population Research Center at the University of Texas at Austin, the University of Queensland, the University of Queensland Library and the reviewers of the monograph manuscript.

1   Introduction

With improvements in and perfection of the medical care for common physical and infectious ailments, more attention is being paid by governments, the media and the academy to illnesses that afflict the mind. The pervasiveness of serious mental illnesses such as schizophrenia and clinical depression in communities across the globe is becoming widely recognised. The increasing impact of dementia, likewise, is being acknowledged as average life spans lengthen across the globe. Chinese societies in mainland China and neighbouring Hong Kong can be considered cases in point, with economic progress leading to significantly increased life expectancy and, so, numbers of dementia cases (Au *et al.* 2010; Ikels 1998; Qiu 2007), as well as a greater focus on quality of life concerns, including mental health (Ramsay 2008).

This book draws attention to the illnesses in question by examining stories recounting Chinese people's experiences of serious mental illness, mostly schizophrenia and related psychoses, but also clinical depression; and family caregiving in dementia. Examination of such accounts, it is believed, can provide great insight into the experience of mental illness and family caregiving in dementia in Chinese societies; more specifically, how this experience is made sense of and represented to others. In examining the stories of mental illness and stories of family caregiving in dementia which originate from a specific cultural community, namely, the Chinese, explication of the salient cultural understandings and forces in play constitutes a key concern of the book.

Research on mental illness and family caregiving in dementia in mainland China and Hong Kong

A body of clinical studies undertaken in mainland China and Hong Kong has drawn attention to the need to take culture into account when developing effective support programs and clinical interventions in mental illness. Pearson has pioneered research into service delivery and rehabilitation, government policy and legislation, and family education and therapy in schizophrenia in mainland China and Hong Kong (Pearson 1995a, 1995b, 1995c, 1996; Pearson and Lam 2002; Pearson and Ning 1997; Pearson and Phillips 1994; Pearson and Tsang 2004; Phillips *et al.* 2002; Wong *et al.* 2003, 2004; Yang and Pearson

2002). Kleinman has pioneered research into the clinical presentation of depression, in particular somatoform disorder, in mainland China, as well as examining stigma in mental illness in mainland China and Hong Kong (Kleinman 1982; Kleinman and Kleinman 1985; Kleinman *et al.* 2011; Lee *et al.* 2006; Lee and Kleinman 2007; Lee *et al.* 2007; Yang and Kleinman 2008). Yip (2007) has focused attention on mainland China in comprehensively examining the epidemiology of mental illnesses, service delivery and rehabilitation, service costs, government policy and legislation, family caregiving and the training of mental health professionals. Meanwhile, Au, Gallagher-Thompson and Ikels have contributed to a comparatively smaller body of clinical studies that draw attention to the role of culture in dementia care and family therapy in mainland China and Hong Kong (Au *et al.* 2009, 2010; Ikels 1998, 2002). Holroyd and Mackenzie have also published more generally in the area of elder care in mainland China and Hong Kong (Holroyd 2001, 2003; Holroyd and Mackenzie 1995, 1997; Mackenzie and Holroyd 1996).

Related humanities research into mental illness and family caregiving in dementia in mainland China and Hong Kong is more limited in amount and generally confined to literary studies of madness. Brassington (1995), Lan (2011), Linder (2011), Rojas (2011) and Yang (2011) have explored the portrayal of mental illness in mainland Chinese literature published in the republican era (1912–1949) and the post-Mao reform period of the late 1970s to date. A relentlessly negative portrayal is found to characterise these literary works. Dikötter (1998) includes some discussion of mental illness in his cultural history of eugenics in mainland China. In this discussion, the strong association between mental illness and heredity in Chinese culture is found to inform government policy and legislation from the republican and communist (1949 onward) periods. Taking a more contemporary focus, Ramsay (2008) has examined the discursive form of psychoeducational brochures and pamphlets put out by public health authorities in mainland China. Mainland Chinese psychoeducational brochures and pamphlets are found to be less biomedicalised and, yet, less empowering for the health consumer when compared to Australian counterparts.

Despite this breadth of clinical and humanities studies, Lee *et al.* (2007, 7) observe that 'Little is known as to how psychopathology is experienced and articulated differently across cultures', in particular, Chinese culture. This book undertakes an in-depth examination of how experiences of mental illness and family caregiving in dementia are articulated within contemporary stories of mental illness and contemporary stories of family caregiving in dementia told by Chinese people living in mainland China and Hong Kong. In so doing, insight is gained into how Chinese culture shapes contemporary stories about two illnesses that afflict the mind and which, at present, are of immense social and clinical importance to mainland China and Hong Kong. The book examines both 'life' (autobiographical and biographical) and 'filmic' (film and television serial drama) stories about the illnesses in question. As such, comparative insights are gained from analysis of contemporary stories told from both 'inside' and 'outside' of the illness experience (Hydén 1997).

The book draws on the perspectives and analytic approaches provided by narrative analysis and cultural studies in order to identify the ways in which Chinese culture shapes the life stories and filmic stories under study. A definition of culture as posed by Ting-Toomey (1999, 9) is embraced:

> First, the term culture refers to a diverse pool of knowledge, shared realities, and clustered norms that constitute the learned systems of meanings in a particular society. Second, these learned systems of meaning are shared and transmitted through everyday interactions among members of the cultural group and from one generation to the next. Third, culture facilitates members' capacity to survive and adapt to their external environment.

Life stories and filmic stories of mental illness and family caregiving in dementia, therefore, will be shaped by the understandings, norms, values and scripts that the storytellers have acquired through being members of a Chinese community. These understandings, norms, values and scripts, in turn, will be conveyed through the stories they tell. Moreover, in telling their stories in ways that are shaped by Chinese culture, the experience of mental illness and family caregiving in dementia, to some degree, is reconciled and made sense of. This can bring a degree of comfort and solace to the storyteller and her or his audience, albeit by necessarily yielding, at times, to the weight of the salient cultural understandings, norms, values and scripts in play.

Culture, stories and illness

The important role of culture in any experience of illness is acknowledged by a body of research to date (Cohen 1998; Hinton and Levkoff 1999; Kleinman *et al.* 2006; Lupton 2003; Squire 2007; Traphagan 2000). Culture informs and dictates people's responses to illness, including views on causation, illness progress and prospective outcomes. It serves as a resource for assigning meaning to an illness, regardless of whether it has been personally experienced.

A principal means by which people fashion and elaborate the meanings assigned to an illness experience is through storytelling (Brody 2003; Lupton 2003; Thomas 2010). This is because, as Pinnegar and Daynes (2007, 4) maintain, stories comprise 'the fundamental unit that accounts for human experience.' Stories, nevertheless, are not incontestable, stable records of human experience (Babrow *et al.* 2005; Bury 2001; Couser 1997; Elliott 2005; Gabriel 2004; Garden 2010; Lieblich *et al.* 1998; Riessman 1993; Shapiro 2011; Thomas 2010). They comprise:

> both less and more than the actual experience: less, in that remembering and writing are selective processes – certain facts are dropped because they are forgotten or because they do not fit the author's narrative design; and more, in that the act of committing experience to narrative form inevitably confers

upon it a particular sequence of events and endows it with a significance that was probably only latent in the original experience.

(Hawkins 1999, 14–15)

Through these processes of selection and conferral, stories provide insight into an experience of illness and its cultural foundations (Bhugra 2006; Charon 2006; Frank 1995, 2010; Garden 2010; Garro and Mattingly 2000a, 2000b; Kleinman 1988; Lupton 2003; Woods 2011). Hydén (1997, 64) states, 'Narrative[1] is one of several cultural forms available to us for conveying, expressing or formulating our experience of illness and suffering. It is also a medium for conveying shared cultural experiences.'

The culturally shaped meanings attached to an illness experience are revealed in how a story rearranges past, present and prospective life events into a temporally and causally coherent sequence (Hurwitz 2004; Hydén and Brockmeier 2008; Riessman 2004) as well as in how the story asserts, refashions and positions emergent identities (Hunt 2000; Hydén 1997; Riessman 2004). The temporal dimension is elementary to any consideration of storytelling (Labov and Waletzky 1997; Ricoeur 1984). Through stories, people locate life events in particular points of time and, in so doing, give form to and provide connection between the seemingly random sequence of events that comprise a person's life (Bakhtin 1981; Bamberg, De Fina and Schiffrin 2007; Brockmeier and Carbaugh 2001; Polanyi 1989; Riessman 1993). This includes the designation of cause in highly disruptive experiences like illness (Bury 1982, 2001; Hydén and Brockmeier 2008). Reordering life events into a temporally and causally coherent sequence not only involves drawing on the past and relating the past to the present, but also involves consideration and contemplation of the future (Clandinan and Connelly 2000; Daiute and Lightfoot 2004; Riessman 2004). Culture can shape when and how temporal and causal connections are made between these life events in a story and guide assessments as to which events are worthy of or suitable for mention (Babrow, Kline and Rawlins 2005; Frank 1995; Garro 2000, 2001; Gergen 2004).

In making sense of a life experience, stories also provide an opportunity for people to engage and cultivate senses of self (Woods 2011). The subjective nature of life experience often leads to considerations of how people locate themselves or others within a series of life events and the extent to which these positionings mediate existing identities or construct new ones (Charon 2006; Cheshire and Ziebland 2005; Harter *et al.* 2005; Hydén and Örulv 2009; Kirmayer 2000). The recursive nature of identity formulation is central to this: stories can both 'present an inner reality to the outside world' and 'shape' new conceptions of self (Lieblich *et al.* 1998, 7). In proclaiming identities, individuals also connect themselves to others in society (Brody 2003; Brockmeier and Carbaugh 2001; Charon 2006; Woods 2011). This may include those who suffer from the same illness. Both real and imagined community attachments, therefore, are often distinguished and affirmed in stories (Hunt 2000; Thornborrow and Coates

2005). Once again, the forms that the asserted or refashioned identities take and the community attachments that they signify will be shaped to a considerable degree by culture (Brody 2003; Hunt 2000).

Cultural meanings are also elaborated through the forms of language used in a story. The link between culture and language is well documented (Ramsay 1997). In research on illness stories, much attention has been given, in particular, to the figurative language characteristically employed in a cultural setting (Garden 2010; Sontag 1989; Wu *et al.* 2004). The communicative power of such language is seen to be derived from its cultural origins, meaningfulness and resonance (Berger 1997; Kleinman 1988). Metaphors, in particular, are of certain value where the aetiological basis of an illness is not well understood, such as in mental illness and dementia, in that they foster a sense of cultural familiarity and offer solace in the face of the unknown. A metaphor commonly employed to represent a person's response to illness in the West is the battle metaphor (Lupton 2003; Sontag 1989). Originally appropriated in the late nineteenth century to characterise the medical response to bacterial infections (Sontag 1989), in more recent times the battle metaphor has come to frame responses to diseases such as cancer, where the aetiological 'enemy' resides within self rather than extraneously. The effective expression of the battle metaphor, Hawkins (1999, 69) states, requires 'an adversary, an enemy "other"[;] ...the patient must feel that the physicians are allies in the battle against disease; and there must be some therapeutic agent or procedure that can act as weaponry.' Frank (2009, 168) views the need for an 'antagonist' in the response to illness as potentially problematic, as it can lead to tensions in self where the battle against the enemy is ultimately fought out. Couser (1997, 45) similarly warns that undue faith in the professional alliance and pharmacotherapeutic armoury 'may encourage the use of "heroic" measures of questionable effectiveness.' The inherent danger is that the adoption of culturally familiar 'metaphors may subvert the project of narrative and come to dominate the sense of self' (Kirmayer 2000, 153). These claims will be tested in the life stories and filmic stories under study.

Analysis of Chinese life stories and filmic stories of mental illness and family caregiving in dementia

Contemporary published life stories and filmic stories of serious mental illness and family caregiving in dementia which are from mainland China and Hong Kong comprise the data sources employed in this book. In line with a number of researchers, the book considers the cultural insights gained from filmic accounts to be as informative as those gained from life accounts (Bartlett *et al.* 1993; Brody 2003; Good and Good 2000; Hydén 1997; Lupton 2003; Miller *et al.* 2005; Roy 2009; Wiltshire 2000). There is deemed to be a potential complementarity between the two forms of stories with content silenced in one form possibly voiced in the other. Filmic stories, for example, tend to more singularly voice the prevailing meta-narrative that circulates in a cultural community, particularly where the meta-narrative is being drawn on for the purpose of broader social and political critique (Bordwell 1985; Branigan 1992; Chouinard 2009; Knight 2006; Lothe 2000; O'Shaughnessy and Stadler 2008; Wedding *et al.* 2005). In light of this, Hydén (1997, 64) has specifically called for studies which illuminate 'the relationship between' the culturally dominant 'grand narratives about illness … and illness narratives constructed by the afflicted themselves.' Such a comparison is undertaken in this book.

The analysis of the life stories and filmic stories under study involves a process of careful reading and scrutiny 'in which patterns of association and contrast are uncovered' (Stewart and Malley 2004, 225). Judgments made in this process are necessarily interpretative (Elliott 2005; Pinnegar and Daynes 2007; Thomas 2010). The process is somewhat complicated by using stories as a data source as this leads the analyst to interpret interpretations, the narrative account itself comprising an interpretation by the storyteller of a life experience (Babrow *et al.*2005; Daiute and Lightfoot 2004; Harter *et al.* 2005; Hawkins 1999; Riessman 1993). The process also involves interpreting what is said and what is not said in the stories (Beck *et al.* 2005; Kirmayer 2000; Riessman 1993; Squire 2005). The *'narrative silences*, the gaps in stories, the unmentioned or unmentionable, as well as the absence of certain stories altogether' are of equal analytic interest as that which is clearly voiced (Harter *et al.* 2005, 13) (original emphasis).

As in any hermeneutic endeavour, alternative interpretations (and so alternative 'realities') will always be possible in relation to the stories analysed (Clandinin and Connelly 2000; Clandinin and Rosiek 2007; Freeman 2001; Lieblich *et al.* 1998; Lupton 2003; Riessman 2000). The aim of the analysis is not 'explanatory completeness or exhaustiveness' in relation to the form and functions of the stories in question (Freeman 2001, 297), but provision of a coherent and plausible account of how culture, as defined above, shapes these stories (Clandinin and Connelly 2000; Clandinin and Rosiek 2007; Harter *et al.* 2005; Riessman 1993). Coherence and plausibility are maintained throughout this book by the adoption of step-by-step methodological frameworks for analysis of the life stories and filmic stories; by making reasoned and grounded associations between the findings for each narrative corpus in formulating a coherent broader analytic picture; by making transparent how analytic interpretations are made through making available multiple illustrative examples from the data; by specification and consideration of the salient contexts in play in the production of the stories in question; and by firmly embedding analytic claims in the existing research literature (Charon 2006; Lieblich *et al.* 1998; Riessman 1993; Thomas 2010).

The Chinese stories under study are sourced from mainland China and Hong Kong. Mainland China and neighbouring Hong Kong (together with nearby Macao), of course, currently make up the People's Republic of China. As corroborated in research from various academic fields of study, Chinese people living in mainland China and Hong Kong share the same fundamental understandings, norms, values and scripts acquired through being members of a Chinese community (Chow 2001; Chung 2001; Holroyd 2003; Lam 2006; Petrus and Wing-chung 2005; Ramsay 2008). These cultural understandings, norms, values and scripts are espoused and upheld throughout a range of life experiences and activities. This would include storytelling in mental illness and in family caregiving in dementia. The book recognises, nevertheless, that Hong Kong possesses a distinct socio-political history in being a British colony for approximately one and a half centuries until joining the People's Republic of China in 1997 (Gray *et al.* 2009). The book, therefore, bears in mind that the regional setting, be it mainland China or Hong Kong, may impact on or nuance the cultural shaping of the stories under study.

Chinese stories of mental illness and family caregiving in dementia

The introductory chapter of the book has established the rationale for the study and outlined the principal research question, namely, how does culture shape stories of mental illness and stories of family caregiving in dementia, both life accounts and filmic accounts, which recount the experiences of Chinese people living in mainland China and Hong Kong? The chapter has delineated the scope of the book and justified the concomitant examination of life stories and filmic stories. The chapter has proffered the definition of culture employed in the book and set out the broad methodological approach followed in analysing the stories under study. It has also acknowledged the potential limitations that attend the use of such data.

Mental illness and dementia both afflict the mind and place a heavy burden on the Chinese family. Mental illness, however, is a functional disorder that usually first appears in young adulthood while dementia is a degenerative disorder commonly associated with old age. Chapters 2 to 4 of the book examine how culture shapes stories of mental illness, with stories of family caregiving in dementia examined in Chapters 5 and 6. Chapter 2 analyses life stories of mainland Chinese people with a mental illness. Published in a mainland Chinese psychoeducational newsletter, the chapter identifies where culture shapes the stories in line with the biomedical agenda and where culture shapes the stories in ways that countermand this agenda. This is demonstrated by reference to the temporal and causal arrangement of life events recounted in the stories, the identities claimed and refashioned therein, and the dominant language forms used. Culturally shaped notions of recovery come to the fore in the chapter. The extent to which cultural shaping of the stories reassures and disempowers the people with a mental illness is also considered.

Chapter 3 of the book analyses life stories of mainland Chinese people who care for a family member with a mental illness. Also published in the mainland Chinese psychoeducational newsletter, the chapter complements Chapter 2 in identifying how culture, at times seemingly 'colluding' with the biomedical agenda while at other times countermanding the biomedical agenda, shapes the stories in question. The chapter discusses the commonalities and differences observed between the life stories written by people with a mental illness and those written by their family caregivers. The issue of cultural stigma, in particular, comes to the fore in the chapter. Once again, the extent to which cultural shaping of the stories reassures and disempowers the family caregivers is considered.

Chapter 4 of the book analyses filmic stories of people with a mental illness recounted in two contemporary mainland Chinese films: *Baober in Love* [恋爱中的宝贝] (2004) and *I Love You* [我爱你] (2002). The chapter compares the ways in which Chinese culture shapes the filmic stories of two women with a mental illness with the ways in which it shapes the life stories analysed in Chapters 2 and 3. This provides an understanding of how culture shapes Chinese people's stories of mental illness told from both inside and outside of the experience. At the same time, the chapter identifies the prevailing meta-narrative of mental illness circulating in Chinese communities, drawn on in the films to critique contemporary mainland Chinese urban life and society allegorically. The chapter considers the discursive connections between the meta-narrative and gender.

Chapter 5 of the book analyses life stories of Chinese people living in Hong Kong, who care for a family member with dementia. Published in an edited work and an autobiographical monograph for the purpose of testimony, the chapter complements the earlier analytic chapters in identifying how culture shapes the stories of family caregiving in dementia, a disease that, like mental illness, afflicts the mind, yet, unlike mental illness, is degenerative and incurable. Particular attention is given to how cultural shaping distinguishes these stories from the mental illness counterparts. Once again, the chapter considers the extent to which cultural shaping of the stories reassures and disempowers the family caregivers. Alongside cultural shaping, the analysis undertaken in the chapter also takes into account the unique socio-political context of Hong Kong.

Chapter 6 of the book analyses filmic stories of family caregiving in dementia recounted in two contemporary mainland Chinese productions: the 2001 film, *Gone is the One Who Held Me Dearest in the World* [世界上最疼我的那个人去了], and the 2005 television serial drama, *Watch for the Happiness* [守望幸福]. As in Chapter 4, the chapter compares the ways in which Chinese culture shapes the stories of two women caring for an elderly family member with dementia with the ways in which it shapes the life stories analysed in Chapter 5. This provides an understanding of how culture shapes Chinese people's stories of family caregiving in dementia told from both inside and outside of the experience. The chapter identifies the prevailing meta-narrative of family caregiving in dementia circulating in Chinese communities, drawn on in the productions to critique contemporary mainland Chinese family life and family relations. The chapter also considers the discursive connections between the meta-narrative and gender.

Chapter 7, the concluding chapter of the book, revisits the issues raised in the introductory chapter in light of the book's analytic findings. The chapter summarises how Chinese culture shapes the life stories and filmic stories of mental illness and family caregiving in dementia which were analysed in

Chapters 2 to 6. The summary draws attention to the interrelationships and interconnections between the key narrative processes that contribute to sense making in these stories: the temporal and causal ordering of life events, the claiming and refashioning of identities, and language use. The chapter considers the issue of the disempowerment and reassurance that can stem from the cultural shaping identified in the stories under study. It also weighs up the methodological strengths and limitations of the book, in particular, the value presented by the use of the complementary data sources, namely, life stories and filmic stories. The chapter contemplates the clinical applications of the book's findings where health services are provided to Chinese clients and identifies potential future research.

2 Life stories of people with a mental illness

This first analytic chapter examines how culture shapes life stories written by mainland Chinese people with a mental illness. The stories are located in the edited volumes *Collected Works on Mental Illness Recovery* [精神疾病康复文集],[1] published in 2000 by the China Science and Technology Publishing House [中国科学技术出版社], and *Since Then My World Has Changed: The Essence of a Decade of 'Mental Illness Recovery News'* [我的世界从此改变—《精神康复报》十年精粹], published in 2007 but with the name of the publisher not stated. Both volumes were edited by Yao Guizhong [姚贵忠], a professor of clinical psychiatry at the Mental Health Research Institute of Beijing University [北京大学精神卫生研究所] and the chief editor of a monthly newsletter published by the Mental Health Research Institute of Beijing University, which is entitled *Mental Illness Recovery News* [精神康复报]. The monthly newsletter, which is distributed across mainland China by way of mental health services and mail order, contains news on recent developments in treatments for mental illness, psychoeducational information written by mental health professionals, as well as a 'letters to the editor' format where people with a mental illness and their family caregivers can submit stories about their own experiences with mental illness. The two edited volumes that supplied the life stories under study in this chapter contain a selection of the stories originally published in the monthly newsletter as well as material written by health professionals, the latter comprising the greater part of the volumes. The life stories and other material comprising the volumes were selected for inclusion by Professor Yao, as editor. *Collected Works on Mental Illness Recovery* contains life stories and other material drawn from the first three years' issues of the monthly newsletter, marking the newsletter's third anniversary of publication, and *Since Then My World Has Changed* contains life stories and other materials drawn from the subsequent seven years' issues of the newsletter, marking the newsletter's tenth anniversary of publication.

Altogether, *Collected Works on Mental Illness Recovery*, a much longer volume (451 pages), supplied 21 life stories, while *Since Then My World Has Changed*, the shorter of the two volumes (166 pages), supplied 12 life stories. Due to the relative closeness of the time periods covered by each of the volumes (July 1997 to July 2000 versus August 2000 to March 2007) it was not expected that there would be any appreciable diachronic variation in how culture shapes the stories in question and this was confirmed in the later analysis. As a consequence, the stories from both volumes were ultimately combined and analysed together as a single 'personal[2] corpus' composed of 33 life stories. The stories range from approximately 400 to 2000 Chinese characters in length (approximating 300 to 1500 English words). They recount personal experiences of severe mental illness, including schizophrenia, bipolar disorder and clinical depression, as follows:

- eighteen schizophrenia stories;
- one clinical depression story;
- two bipolar disorder stories;
- twelve 'mental illness' (diagnostic name unspecified) stories.

The vast majority of the stories that did not specify a diagnostic name for the mental illness in question speak of psychotic experiences in their narrative content. Experiences of schizophrenia/psychotic illness, therefore, dominate the narrative corpus.

Nine authors of the stories in question were identifiable as women, seven as men, with the remainder (seventeen) of undeterminable gender. The 'living status' of the authors varied as follows:

- seventeen 'adult-children', that is, adults living at home with their parents, comprising five women, four men and eight of undeterminable gender;
- three spouses, comprising one woman and two men;
- one independent single, that is, person living independently, comprising one man.
- twelve of undeterminable living status, comprising three women and nine of undeterminable gender.

Thus, where gender is determinable, there appears an approximately even split in representation of women's and men's stories. Given the large number of stories about schizophrenia/psychotic illness and given that over 90 per cent of people with schizophrenia in mainland China live at home with their families (Phillips 1993; Ran *et al.* 2005; Yip 2007), it is likely that the vast majority of the 12 authors of undeterminable living status are adult-children. Thus, the stories of adult-children appear to dominate the narrative corpus.

The socioeconomic and class backgrounds of the authors of the life stories are not immediately evident, due to the nature of the data as published, largely de-identified accounts. While many authors recount the severe financial pressures they face, the fact that they have been able to access formal mental health services when around 80 per cent of people with a serious mental illness remain untreated in mainland China (Lee and Kleinman 2007; Pearson 1996; Ran *et al.* 2005), and considering the educational and vocational backgrounds of authors as recounted in their stories, it is unlikely that they belong to impoverished families or to the rural-dwelling peasant class. Based on the content of their stories, most authors appear to live in small to medium towns or large urban centres.

According to Thornborrow and Coates, the life stories under study would constitute 'public' stories, due to their institutional means of dissemination and public readership. As such, they may possess features that distinguish them from the 'private' stories of day-to-day conversation or interview (Thornborrow and Coates 2005, 6). There are, of course, potential limitations in using such stories. Firstly, they have been selected for publication by the editor of the monthly newsletters and then the editor of the anniversary volumes, Yao Guizhong in both instances. It is likely that this has been undertaken keeping in mind the psychoeducational intent of these publications. Stories advocating practices that run counter to the goals of psychoeducation or which are overly critical of formal mental health services may have been edited out. This issue relates more broadly to that of intended readership and its influence on both the writing of and publication of public stories (Elliott 2005; Frank 1995; Garro and Mattingly 2000b; McKay and Bonner 2002). The impact of the psychoeducational context of publication of the life stories examined in this chapter, therefore, becomes an important consideration in the ensuing analysis of how culture shapes these stories.

A second potential limitation is that the readership of the newsletter where the stories were originally published comprises a 'community' in the sense of a group of people with similar life experiences. Namely, they have faced mental illness and sought treatment for it at a hospital mental health unit. In functioning as a support group, this community may have developed prescriptions as to what constitutes a 'good' story of mental illness (Ayometzi 2007; Brody 2003; Feldman 2001; Garden 2010; Garro and Mattingly 2000a; Shapiro 2011). Japp (2005, 55) states that 'Personal stories are vital to healing across a spectrum of health and illness experiences, but as stories migrate into public dialogue, they can no longer be understood solely as personal expressions of experience.' The stories in question, therefore, may as much recount a preferred experience of mental illness as a truly personal one, this preferred experience having evolved as life stories have been told and retold in the newsletter forum. Nevertheless, regardless of the extent to which the stories told before have moulded the subsequent stories (a subcultural shaping, if you will), cultural shaping, which is the key concern of this book, would remain in evidence.

A third potential limitation of the stories in question is the potential for 'ghost-writing' or co-authorship. Particularly in the case of people with a severe mental illness, some assistance in the writing of their life stories may have come from, for example, family members or health professionals. While this cannot be wholly ruled out, the subsequent analysis undertaken in Chapter 3 does reveal clear differences between the stories written by people with a mental illness and their family caregivers, some, in fact, representing contradictory understandings and viewpoints. Similarly, experiences of medical intervention by health professionals are not always positively represented. This suggests that co-authorship by family caregivers or health professionals was likely minimal and had little impact on the narrative corpus taken as a whole. Regardless, cultural shaping would remain in evidence in co-authored stories.

These potential limitations attending the use of public stories, nevertheless, need to be viewed in light of the advantages that they present (Elliott 2005; O'Brien and Clark 2010). The stories have been freely written in the people's own time for inclusion in the monthly psychoeducational newsletter. They have had ample time for reflection on and consideration of their experiences of mental illness. As such, they remain unaffected by any contexts of interview and by any potential influence or leading of narrative content or structure by interviewers through their preconceived agenda (Cortazzi 1993; Freeman 2004; Hydén 1995; O'Brien and Clark 2010).

Analytic procedure

This chapter adopts the methodological approach followed by Hemsley *et al.* (2007), Öhman and Söderberg (2004), Pejlert (2001) and Stoltz *et al.* (2006), amongst others, to analyse the illness experience as recounted in a corpus of illness stories. The approach, described as 'phenomenological hermeneutic' in that it involves *interpreting* narrative accounts in order to come to an understanding of the *meaning* of the recounted illness *experience*, is a useful starting point for the task at hand since it provides a systematic means of identifying and constructing a common, shared experience of illness from a collection of related life stories (Elliott 2005; Mishler 1995). The approach is particularly worthwhile, it is believed, because the analytic steps that a researcher needs to document when adopting this approach mirror those undertaken in the analyst's mind as she or he engages in a recursive process of careful reading in order to uncover the threads of connection and essential meanings existing at the different layers of a story (see Chapter 1). The approach also accommodates the examination of a corpus of life stories in order to identify where 'each new life story appears to confirm the main elements of the previous stories' (Elliott 2005, 40), as undertaken in the current chapter.

Specifically, the researcher begins by documenting a 'naïve understanding' gained from an initial reading of the stories under study (Öhman and Söderberg 2004, 399). This equates to a first impression of the stories being told: what Stoltz *et al.* (2006, 597) call 'a first surface conjecture'. This is followed by documenting the results of a detailed sentence-by-sentence analysis of the linguistic and semantic structures that comprise the text. In this stage, specific thematic and linguistic features are identified, illustrated and systematically organised (Stoltz *et al.* 2006). In so doing, the formative 'parts of and patterns in the text' are exposed (Öhman and Söderberg 2004, 399). Numerous textual examples, transcribed in Chinese with English translations in this book, make primary narrative data available to the reader and are employed to illustrate the means by which structural groupings are achieved and associations between groupings are made (Riessman 1993). These illustrative examples provide the reader with a degree of access to the language and content of the stories in question, given that complete transcripts of these stories cannot be reproduced in this book. The examples also provide transparency as to how interpretations are made in the subsequent stage of the analysis, transparency constituting an essential element in analyses of this type (see Chapter 1).

The final analytic stage involves the formulation of a 'comprehensive understanding' of the stories under study, based on the research question driving the study (Öhman and Söderberg 2004, 399). In this stage, a critical analysis of what is being said in the stories and why it is being said this way is undertaken. This usually entails consideration of context, the said and unsaid, as well as the relevant existing research literature (Stoltz *et al.* 2006). Relevant thematic and linguistic features identified and illustrated in the preceding stage are drawn on in this final analytic stage to examine and account for, in terms of the current chapter, how culture shapes the mainland Chinese life stories of mental illness.

Analysis of personal life stories of mental illness

Naïve understanding

Taken together, the life stories under study reveal close identification of the person with her or his illness. People are defined by their illness, with a sense of community developing around those who suffer from like illness. A salient element in the experience of mental illness is loss: financial cost, future uncertainty, diminished social status and diminished self-worth. These losses can lead to contemplation of or attempts at suicide. For most, however, the personal challenges that mental illness presents lead to reflection on the means of support that is drawn on to face and overcome these challenges. Principal sources of support and reliance recounted in the stories under study include self, family, health professionals and society in general. None of these sources are overridingly dominant. Some look to self; some depend heavily on their families, in particular their parents; some look to health professionals for guidance in life; while others find solace in the society around them. In facing the challenges presented by mental illness people reveal a prevailing sense of hope or positivity toward existing circumstances and the future. Drawing on their preferred sources of support and embracing a positive outlook play an important part in people with a mental illness achieving their primary goal in 'recovery': for some developing a sense of personal achievement and self-efficacy; for others re-engagement with society and fulfilling cultural expectations to contribute to society, mostly through engaging in productive work. Despite the psychoeducational context of publication of the stories in question, medical intervention informs the experience of mental illness only for some, who overwhelmingly view medication compliance as integral to 'recovery'. Nevertheless, medical intervention is rarely unproblematic, frequently involving pharmacotherapeutic failure, residual symptomatology or untoward medication side-effects. The most commonly accepted aetiological basis to mental illness recounted in the stories is psychosocial factors, with biogenetic factors rarely entertained. This, too, occurs despite the psychoeducational context of publication of the stories in question and the documented hegemony of the biomedical explanatory model of mental illness in mainland Chinese mental health circles (Kleinman and Kleinman 1985; Pearson 1995a; Phillips 1993; Ran *et al.* 2005; Tseng 1986).

Sentence level structural analysis

Analysis of the sentence level linguistic and semantic features of the life stories under study reveals the following salient themes and subthemes pertaining to the personal experience of mental illness (Table 2.1). They are discussed and illustrated in the following pages.

Table 2.1 Salient themes and subthemes in mainland Chinese personal stories of mental illness

Theme	Subtheme
Embracing of 'illness identity'	Self identified by illness Identification with 'illness community'
Mental illness causes loss	Financial cost of mental illness Loss of future expectations Loss of self-worth and social status Loss leading to contemplation of or attempt at suicide
Foci of support and reliance	Importance of self-reliance Dependence on family Reliance on professional guidance Support from broader society
Maintenance of hope and positivity	Value of hope and positivity Positive reinterpretation
Social basis to 'recovery'	Importance of social contact and engagement Contribution to society Value of work
Biomedical intervention	Non-compliance leads to relapse Pharmacotherapeutic failure, residual symptomatology and medication side-effects
Explanatory models of mental illness	Mental illness has a psychosocial aetiology Mental illness has a biomedical aetiology Mental illness is caused by malnutrition

Embracing of 'illness identity'

Many of the stories in question possess statements suggesting an intimate and defining relationship between the person's sense of self and the mental illness that he or she suffers from. Personal subjectivity is 'named' by the illness through statements, commonly made at the outset of a story, such as 'I am a schizophrenia sufferer'[3] [我是一位精神分裂症患者] (Text 1, Yao 2000, 312) and 'I am a bipolar disorder sufferer' [我是一名躁郁症患者] (Text 20, Yao 2000, 366). The personhood of the authors is seemingly closely linked to their illness and, as such, to the prevailing social view of the illness which can come to define them (Wisdom *et al.* 2008).

In a number of these stories, membership of a broader 'illness community' is expressed by means of collectively worded statements such as 'We are all ill-fated and very unfortunate mentally-disabled people' [我们是一个个命运坎坷，又是十分不幸的精神残疾人] (Text 18, Yao 2000, 353); 'We mental illness sufferers all have consciences, but when we suffer a breakdown we also can be scary' [我们精神病人都很有良心，但犯起毛病来也是可怕的] (Text 28, Yao 2007, 20). Membership of this community can provide a sense of connection and belonging, as well as an avenue of grass-roots support, for people with a mental illness.

> Among fellow sufferers, and through our contact with health care workers, we have formed a microcosm of life. In this environment I have experienced care and concern, felt understanding and solace, felt the confidence to overcome difficulties together, and felt the courage to live as well as the value of life.
> [在病友之间，在与医护人员的交往中间，我们形成了生命的一个微型环境，在这个环境里，我感受到了关怀和爱护，感到了理解和慰藉，感受到了共同战胜困难的信心，还有生活的勇气和价值。]
>
> (Text 10, Yao 2000, 338)
>
> I wish the whole world of fellow sufferers, finding company in their misery, to recover as I have.
> [祝天下同病相怜的病友都像我一样康复。]
>
> (Text 30, Yao 2007, 25)

The claiming of an illness identity is also, at times, voiced alongside expressions of lament for the challenges that mental illness bring. Mental illness in mainland China, as in many Confucian-heritage societies, 'disembodies' the individual by removing 'the ability to function not only as a social, but as a cultural entity' (Traphagan 2000, 8). As such, the individual is viewed as 'burdensome and embarrassing to the most immediate group to which he belongs – the household' (Traphagan 2000, 153). For some people with a mental illness, remorse over the emotional and material pressures placed on their families due to their disembodiment may be attenuated and accommodated by seeking refuge in the illness identity, which supplies a culturally coherent explanation for apparent underachievement and a high level of dependency (Hunt 2000; Kleinman 1982; Kleinman and Kleinman 1985).

> I have become a person living at the bottom of society .... My hallucinations and delusions are profuse ... but I could speak forever about my parents' love for me. I am a schizophrenia sufferer.
> [我成了生活在社会最底层的人 ... 我的幻觉妄想是丰富的 ... 而爸爸妈妈对我的爱却永远讲不完. 我是一位精神分裂症患者]
>
> (Text 1, Yao 2000, 311–312)

> I am an unfortunate mental illness sufferer, but fortunately, I have a very warm home.
> [我是一个不幸的精神病患者, 但幸运的是, 我有一个非常温暖的家.]
>
> (Text 32, Yao 2007, 28)

Mental illness causes loss

A sense of loss marks many of the stories. The specific experiences that give rise to a sense of loss vary, with no particular issue notably dominating. Some stories speak of material losses associated with the financial pressures of the health care costs in treating the mental illness. In Mao's People's Republic (1949–1976), urban dwellers working for state-owned industries and the government received free or heavily subsidised health care. Since 1978, economic reforms and fundamental changes in employment modes and arrangements have resulted in health care, for the most part, being provided on a user-pays basis (Kohrman 2005; Yip 2007).

> With a monthly wage of 600 Yuan[4], plus Mother's retirement pension of 500 Yuan, mother and son need to rely on each other to get by and bear the burden of the 600 Yuan cost of medication every month.
> [每月有600元的工资, 加上母亲500元的退休金, 母子俩相依为命, 负担着每月600元的药费.]
>
> (Text 6, Yao 2000, 332)

> At the time I received sick-leave pay of 21 Yuan 7 Jiao[5] per month. Mental turmoil and economic impoverishment made me sink into an abyss of suffering.
> [当时我每月拿的是21元7角的长病假工资. 精神上的错乱和经济上的贫困使我陷入了痛苦的深渊.]
>
> (Text 18, Yao 2000, 354)

The financial pressure can be particularly marked in an illness like schizophrenia. This is because it commonly impacts just as the person is entering the workforce or has only recently entered the workforce; and just when the person's primary caregivers are usually planning to leave the workforce or have recently retired.

Loss of confidence and certainty in future goals and expectations is a feature for some. This can be particularly troublesome in settings like mainland China where there are strong cultural expectations to seek and maintain reliable employment, marry, have children, and take care of parents in their retirement.

> Thinking about the future, there really are many uncertain factors. My parents are old, but in my present circumstances I am not fit to take care of others. I'm steadily getting older, and so I have to consider the problem of getting married and settling down.
> [想一想未来, 的确有很多不确定的因素, 爸爸妈妈都老了, 而我现在这种情况还缺不了别人的照顾. 年龄逐渐增大, 成家立业的问题也不能不考虑.]
>
> (Text 6, Yao 2000, 332)

> Falling ill clearly increased my sense of disappointment in life. I lost all confidence in my life outlook.
> [患病使我对生活的失望感明显加强, 对人生的前途没有信心.]
>
> (Text 17, Yao 2000, 352)

The effects of mental illness can also cause some to lose their sense of self-worth, unable to fulfil personal and cultural expectations of life:

> I have lost a lot because of my disease. To date I have no children to bring me happiness. I live in a household that is wholly dull and silent. I have no thriving career and, as far as I'm concerned, master's and doctoral degrees remain an unattainable dream.
> [因为疾病我失去了许多. 到目前为止, 我没有子女给我带来的快乐, 我充分的体验着家庭的平淡与宁静. 事业上也没有蒸蒸日上, 硕士与博士学位, 对我来说是一种不可企及的梦.]
>
> (Text 10, Yao 2000, 338)

> Thinking of the onset of my illness, I was just like a human vegetable. I didn't possess even the most basic capabilities to take care of myself …. Everyone knew I had gone mad. Those teachers who had taught me in the past, on seeing me, would shun me in fear of getting into trouble. Those who had once professed to be my best friends and classmates came to view me with contempt. And along the road, a group of six or seven-year-old children called out 'madman' while chasing after me, throwing small pebbles at me.
> [想到自己发病时就像植物人一样, 连最基本的自理能力都没有 … 所有的人都知道我是疯子了, 那些曾经教导过我的老师见了我就避之唯恐不及; 曾经自称是我最好的朋友、同学, 开始对我白眼相加了. 一路上, 一群六七岁大的孩子一边喊着"疯子"一边追赶着我, 将小石子丢到我身上.]
>
> (Text 22, Yao 2007, 2–3)

People with a mental illness come to view themselves as 'a person from the bottom of society' [社会最底层的人] (Text 1, Yao 2000, 311), who 'deeply feels one's own inadequacy' [深感自己不足] (Text 13, Yao 2000, 342). This can lead to contemplation of suicide: 'I once thought about ending my life' [我曾想过放弃生命] (Text 11, Yao 2000, 339); or attempts at the same: 'Because of this I once attempted suicide' [为此我曾自杀过] (Text 17, Yao 2000, 352); '[this] drove me to take up a knife and slash my wrists on many occasions' [促使我多次拿起刀割脉] (Text 29, Yao 2007, 22).

Foci of support and reliance

People with a mental illness require sources of support and reliance to aid them to adapt to or to overcome the aforementioned challenges that they must face in their daily lives. The sources of support and dependence recounted in the life stories under study include self, family, health professionals and broader society. Comparatively speaking, across the narrative corpus, family is least resonant (nine texts) and self most resonant (fourteen texts).

The resonance of self as the focus of support and reliance is possibly surprising, given the family/social orientation in Chinese culture (Bakken 2000; Ng *et al.* 2008b; Yip 2007). One may have expected a stronger 'other-orientation' in relation to this phenomenon. The psychoeducational context of publication of the stories in question may be a factor here, in that it would likely be deemed favourable by health authorities for people with a mental illness to develop a sense of independence in action and insight into the circumstances of their illnesses. Moreover, the concept of independence in the Chinese cultural context does not signify total self-sufficiency and financial autonomy as it would in the West, but being able to actively and gainfully contribute to household duties and finances as is deemed appropriate to a person's age and gender (Pearson 1996; Traphagan 2000).[6]

Additionally, the illness identity so resonant across the corpus and the sense of illness community that this connotes would suggest that the phenomenon of self-reliance may not merely encompass individual, single-handed action but also support from and reliance on the community of fellow illness sufferers. Indeed, this is suggested by the following passages where self-reliance is presented as a salient feature of the authors' personal ethos in facing up to mental illness, yet it is addressed collectively in terms of a perceived illness community.

> We need to take heed of the words of a wise man: the strong work toward their own goals while the weak take on the opinions of those around them. We need to be strong. We need to work toward our own goal, namely overcoming mental illness.
> [大家要记住一位哲人的话: 强者, 为自己的目标活着; 弱者, 为周围的舆论 所左右. 我们要做个强者, 我们要为自己的目标而活着, 我们的目标是战胜精神病.]
>
> (Text 4, Yao 2000, 321–322)

> What I would like to tell you is that the person who will rescue you from your fate is not another person, but yourself.
> [我想告诉大家的是, 拯救你命运的人不是别人, 就是你自己.]
>
> (Text 14, Yao 2000, 343)

A happy life can only be brought about by relying on your own efforts and by making a change from putting the blame on others to drawing encouragement from your own strengths.
[幸福生活是要靠自己劳动来创造的, 把怨天尤人变为鞭策自己的力量.]

(Text 24, Yao 2007, 6)

Direct references to self-achievement, while atypical, do occur in the corpus:

I believe that the making of who I am today to a large extent is a product of my own efforts. [我认为弄成今天这个样子, 在很大程度上是自己造成的.]

(Text 21, Yao 2000, 372).

Another rejects 'leading a "parasitic" life' [过着"寄生"的生活] (Text 33, Yao 2007, 105) of total financial dependence on the family.

The efforts individuals must make in facing the challenges presented by mental illness, either alone or as part of their illness community, are commonly recounted by drawing on metaphors of long-term 'struggle' and 'battle'. Also documented in Western illness stories (see Chapter 1), the mainland Chinese metaphors possess clear historical and political resonances, adopting language stemming from China's resistance to Japanese invasion in the 1930s and 1940s and the subsequent communist revolution characterised by successive ideological campaigns and movements. A person's fight against mental illness, therefore, is located within a wider system of cultural meaning and reference (Kleinman 1988) that embodies his or her invested effort as 'heroic' (Bury 2001; Carney 2004).

One must also triumph over the torment of illness. This is truly adding even more difficulty to the challenge. But, as long as one perseveres – while others take five years, I may take ten years. As the saying goes 'persistence is victory.'
[还要战胜疾病的折磨, 真是难上加难. 但是只要有恒心, 别人用五年我用十年, 俗话说"坚持就是胜利".]

(Text 12, Yao 2000, 341)

One can completely triumph over schizophrenia. Of course, the most important thing is sufferers themselves must have a deep passion for living and cherish life. In the face of a life catastrophe, a person who takes responsibility for his or her own life will surely mount a spirited counterattack and ultimately triumph over disaster.
[精神分裂症是完全可以被战胜的. 当然, 最重要的还是患者本人一定要热爱生活, 珍惜生命, 一个对自己生命负责的人在人生的灾难面前一定会奋起反击, 最终战胜灾难.]

(Text 25, Yao 2007, 14)

Resonance of the family as the focus of support in the life stories is unsurprising, given the fundamental role that the family plays in Chinese culture in terms of provision of support and caregiving, particularly in illness. This is well documented in relation to mental illness in mainland China (Pearson and Lam 2002; Ramsay 2008; Yang and Pearson 2002; Yip 2007). A characteristic of references to family support and reliance in these stories is the depth of gratitude and feeling created by the family members', mostly parents', actions.

> My hallucinations and delusions are profuse. At present I can still prattle on for several hours; but I could speak forever about my parents' love for me.
> [我的幻觉妄想是丰富的, 现在我还可以滔滔不绝地讲上几小时, 而爸爸妈妈对我的爱却永远讲不完.]
>
> (Text 1, Yao 2000, 312)

> Mother, who gave birth to me, who raised me, who loves me, who saved me; ah, you drew on every drop of blood in your body to cast your daughter's road to recovery. You drew on your great maternal love to rescue your daughter's dying soul. You have shone brilliant sunlight onto me. You have caused me to enter the seasons of joy. You have taken me to clear and sunny skies.
> [生我, 养我, 爱我, 救我的妈妈啊, 您用滴滴心血浇铸了女儿的康复之路, 您用伟大的母爱挽救了女儿濒死的灵魂, 是您撒给我灿烂的阳光, 是您令我走进缤纷的季节, 您为我撑起了一片晴朗的天空.]
>
> (Text 19, Yao 2000, 366)

For these people, parents encompass the sole form of interpersonal contact and sole focus of leisure activity. Nevertheless, the high degree of integration of these people's daily lives into those of their parents would still constitute independence in the Chinese cultural context as long as the person with a mental illness actively and gainfully contributes to the household duties and finances, as noted earlier.

The resonance of health professionals as the focus of support is unsurprising, given the psychoeducational context of publication of the stories. This support commonly extends beyond the proffering of professional advice to structured guidance and direction.

> The most important thing is to fit in with the psychiatrist and to actively communicate with the psychologist. As I say, 'one hand holds the hand of the psychiatrist and the other hand holds the hand of the psychologist'.
> [最重要的是跟精神科医生配合, 跟心理医生主动沟通, 按我的话说就是"一手拉着精神科医生的手, 一手拉着心理医生的手".]
>
> (Text 2, Yao 2000, 313)

> Thinking back over my seven years of suffering in the past and looking now at these seventeen years of happiness, I would like to wholeheartedly thank

the rehabilitation centre[7], this fine organisation of such benefit to the people. It gives mental illness sufferers a new lease on life.
[回想过去痛苦的7年, 看看如今这幸福的17年, 我衷心感谢工疗站这个为民造福的好组织, 使精神病患者重获新生.]

(Text 18, Yao 2000, 355)

During the out-patient check-up I told my doctor about my progress. My doctor was very pleased, at the same time proposing even higher requirements of me.
[门诊复查的时候, 我把我的进步跟医生说了, 医生也很满意, 同时对我提出了更高的要求.]

(Text 21, Yao 2000, 373)

The final focus of support for people with a mental illness is society in general. The 'other-orientation' characterising Chinese culture has already been noted. It has been argued that the phenomenon of other-orientation may inform self-reliance in the stories, with the immediate social group in this circumstance being the 'illness community'. However, there is also reference in the narrative corpus to people gaining support from and relying on society more broadly, that is, general members of or bodies located in the person's local community or the wider nation. Here, people speak emotively of society's 'concern' [关心], 'guidance' [开导], 'encouragement' [鼓励] and 'warmth' [温暖] (Text 5, Yao 2000, 323); society's 'care' [关怀] and 'consideration' [照顾] (Text 18, Yao 2000, 355); and society's 'voice of praise' [赞扬声] (Text 21, Yao 2000, 373). In these stories, social support and reliance take on remedial, moral and material dimensions.

Yet, as soon as I chatted with normal people, even though we wouldn't talk about my illness but would merely chat about everyday matters – or if I simply listened to them chatting – their words would, like a cleaning agent, wash away the residual symptoms in my mind. Over time this proved beneficial to my recovery from my illness.
[可我一和正常人聊天, 尽管不是聊自己的病, 只是聊周围的事情, 或者只是听人家聊, 正常人的话就像洗涤剂那样清扫我脑子里的"类妄想", 久而久之对病的恢复会有好处的.]

(Text 4, Yao 2000, 321)

When I first fell ill I always observed other people's attitude toward me and what I saw was only well-intentioned concern and kind greetings. I never personally saw or heard anyone say anything bad about me. When other people spoke to me they were careful in their choice of words, fearing they could harm me … I love the extended family that is our society.
[我患病之初, 总观察别人对我的态度, 而我看到的只是善意的关心和问候, 从未亲见或听说有谁说我什么不好, 别人对我讲话时用词都很谨慎, 就怕伤害到我 … 我爱我们的社会大家庭.]

(Text 15, Yao 2000, 348, 350)

Disregarding the disruption to work, my workplace still reimbursed me for all my medical expenses. At year-end they also came to visit us workers who were experiencing difficulties and presented us with some cash support. This made me feel the warmth of the extended family that is our society.

[工作上的损失不算，单位还给我报销全部的医药费，年终还来看望我们这些困难职工，并送上慰问金，使我感到社会大家庭的温暖。]

(Text 28, Yao 2007, 21)

Maintenance of hope and positivity

Maintaining a hopeful and positive outlook, despite the losses that attend mental illness, features in many of the life stories. Considered by Western psychoeducational research to be effective coping responses in mental illness (Stein *et al.* 2007), hope and positivity, coupled with goal-setting behaviour, comprise the preferred response in Chinese culture to challenging circumstances such as mental illness (Pearson and Phillips 1994; Phillips 1993; Xiong *et al.* 1994; Yang and Pearson 2002). Hope and positivity are future oriented (Lam *et al.* 2011), and buoyed in the life stories by the person's focus of support and reliance, namely, self, illness community, family, health professional and society, as discussed above.

But I believe that invested effort will always receive a payback in return; that tenacious perseverance will surely overcome illness. And I wish that fellow sufferers of forms of mental illness will join me in efforts to move forward toward the better future that lies ahead.

[但我想，付出总会有回报，顽强的毅力一定会战胜病痛. 我也祝愿和我一样患有精神方面病痛的病友们，和我一起向着美好的未来努力前行。]

(Text 2, Yao 2000, 313)

Looking back, I have already walked along too many uneven paths. What can one do? Life does not accept tears and weakness. In front of me lies just one path: I have no choice but to build confidence and bravely continue.

[回头看看，自己已经走过太多不平坦的路，有什么办法呢，生活不相信眼泪和懦弱，面前只有一条路，我只能建立信心，勇敢地走下去。]

(Text 6, Yao 2000, 332)

However, we only live once. The dense fog will eventually disperse and, so long as we're still alive, we'll eventually be greeted by a bright and sunny sky. I believe that everyone experiences illness. I am much more fortunate than people suffering from cancer or uraemia. There are still medications to treat my illness and the possibility of a complete recovery.

[然而生命只有一次，迷雾终将散去. 只要还活着，我们终会迎来阳光灿烂的天空. 我想：人吃五谷哪有不生病的，比起患癌症、尿毒症的病人，我幸运多了，还有药物可医治，还有痊愈的可能。]

(Text 23, Yao 2007, 4)

The past and present are also 'positively reinterpreted' at times, with the challenges faced in mental illness re-evaluated as 'a learning or growth experience' (Lefley 1996, 116). The overcoming of such challenges is evidence of attainment of a high degree of personal resilience and self-efficacy (Hawkins 1999; Lam *et al.* 2011).

> What life has bestowed upon me [mental illness] is something that I do not want at all. Yet I view it as a precious gift because it has made me accept the test of life and given my life a reconveyed sense of meaning.
> [生命所赐予我的是我并不想要的东西，然而，我将其视为一个珍贵的礼物，因为它使我接受了人生的考验，给我的生命重新赋予了含义.]
>
> (Text 10, Yao 2000, 338)

> That period of time when I deferred my studies [due to mental illness] has passed by. When I look back now, I find that those were idyllic days, even though there remains a slight hint of sadness. Since then I have been through many days of despondency, even more so than back then, however I am no longer depressed nor full of sorrow. I am much calmer than before and much more relaxed. I suppose that life is a never-ending textbook.
> [休学的那段日子我度过了. 当我现在回首的时候，我觉得那段日子是一幅田园诗景，尽管有点淡淡的忧伤. 在那之后，我还经历了许多比那更为惆怅的日子，然而，我已经不再忧郁、不再悲伤，我变得比以前更为平静、更为豁达. 我想说，生活是一本读不完的教科书.]
>
> (Text 14, Yao 2000, 343)

Social basis to 'recovery'

In many of the life stories there is a strong social basis to the definition of 'recovery' from mental illness (Lysaker *et al.* 2010). People place great value on re-establishing everyday social contact and re-engaging in social activity as measures of their return to a healthy mental state and their 'return to society' [回归社会; 重返社会].[8] Self-meaning, here, is actualised through social contact as well as through a person's ability to contribute to society (or nation) through productive work or similar activities. Thus, for these people, the gains of recovery are less about feelings of improved self-efficacy and personal achievement per se and more about how recovery enables them to be able to fulfil the cultural expectations of what constitutes a whole and valuable member of the community and the state (Kleinman *et al.* 2011; Traphagan 2000).

> At the time, social contact was what I feared the most, yet it was also something most helpful in the recovery from my condition. What's more, it also constitutes the final stage of and goal of our recovery. Then, bit by bit I got used to interacting with people and trying to take the initiative to talk with people. Offering my heart in good faith I successfully gained everyone's approval. Nowadays I no longer fear there being more strangers

around. What's more, having joined the workforce I have assimilated back into society.

[社交是我当时觉得最怕却也是对我病情恢复最有帮助的事, 并且也是我们康复的最后阶段和目的 … 我便一点一滴地适应与人的交往, 尝试主动与人说话, 捧出自己真诚的心, 便很成功地赢得了大家的喜爱. 现在生人再多我也不怕了, 并且参加了工作, 我又融入了社会.]

(Text 15, Yao 2000, 349–350)

In the wake of changes in my surroundings and improvement in my social adaptation, especially the experience I gained from working, I slowly cast off my unhealthy state of mind … I gradually came to understand that the value of life is raised through commitment. The more things you do for society, the happier you will be. Even though we are remunerated for working and this remuneration also guarantees our standard of living, even more important is that work allows us to build a bridge for connecting to society and other people. Creating such a 'bridge' greatly enriches our life and strengthens our personality. Pity the person who is separated from society and the people … More mentally ill people can have the opportunity to return to society, return to the people.

[随着环境的改变, 社会适应能力的增强, 特别是工作给我带来的经验, 我慢慢地摆脱了不健康的心绪 … 我逐渐领悟到, 生命的价值在奉献中升华. 你为社会多做了一些事情, 你自己就会更加愉快. 虽然我们的工作都是有报酬的, 这种报酬亦保证了我们的生活水平, 但更重要的是工作使我们与社会及他人架起了一座联系的桥梁, 这种"桥梁"的建立, 极大地丰富了我们的人生, 健全了我们的人格. 一个脱离社会和人群的人是可怜的 … 更多的精神病人能够有机会回到社会中, 回到人群中.]

(Text 17, Yao 2000, 352–353)

Biomedical intervention

The 'voice of biomedicine' in any form of mental health discourse can be viewed as one which enunciates

a highly biomedicalised conception of mental illness. This conception views imbalances in the body's neurochemistry as the aetiological basis for mental illness, and promotes the timely use of medication and adjunct therapies as the key to alleviation of clinical signs.

(Ramsay 2008, 109)

The biomedical voice has somewhat low positive resonance in the life stories under study, despite their psychoeducational context of publication. Unequivocally positive accounts of biomedical intervention are few, with the seemingly negative subthemes of untoward medication side-effects, niggling residual symptomatology and outright pharmacotherapeutic failure more commonly in evidence (Lam *et al.* 2011). The common subtheme of 'non-compliance leads to relapse', while not strictly negative in tone, nevertheless voices the authoritative (biomedical) imperative (Ng *et al.* 2011). This imperative emphasises strict compliance with the pharmacotherapeutic regime prescribed by the health professional rather than the positive outcomes of pharmacotherapy. As such, medication is rarely spoken of as bringing positive gains to the life of the person with a mental illness but as something that must be taken as directed by the health professional lest the person falls ill again. Thus, while biomedical intervention frames the pathway to recovery for many, it is by no means an unequivocally pleasant experience.

In 1996 I met a boyfriend who wanted to get married straight away and have a baby. I was worried that because I was taking medication, I may give birth to a disabled child, so I again stopped taking my medication in early 1997. After I stopped my medication, my condition relapsed once again and more seriously than before. Not only did I get hallucinations, but I also had suicidal thoughts of lying on the railway tracks or jumping off a building. Mother took me to hospital again for treatment where the doctor made me take Risperdal and Prozac. The results were not obvious after having taken them for nearly two months, and my menstruation also became irregular.
[1996年, 我结识了一个男朋友, 对方迫切要求结婚生孩子. 我担心由于用药, 生育残疾儿, 于1997年初又停药了. 停药后病情再度复发, 而且比以前还厉害, 不但有幻觉, 而且还想死, 向卧轨、跳楼. 妈妈又领我到医院诊治, 医生让我服用维思通和百优解, 服了近两个月, 效果不明显, 而且月经也不正常了.]

(Text 3, Yao 2000, 314)

This stay in hospital lasted five months. Initially I was injected with sedative and later changed to oral Clozapine. Both were ineffective. In the end insulin shock therapy was used and my condition gradually stabilised after more than 40 days of treatment, yet there were still some residual auditory hallucinations …. I resumed my studies, but 14 or 15 hours of every day were spent sleeping and after waking up I still felt all washed out …. Because of long-term use of Clozapine, two years after I was discharged from hospital my white blood cell count suddenly dropped. I had to change my medication and started on Fluanxol. At the time I was just getting ready to return home to celebrate the New Year and the doctor said that I was likely to completely recover this time. I was very pleased. However, in fact it turned out completely the opposite. I reacted very severely to Fluanxol, feeling agitated and experiencing a large number of auditory hallucinations. What's more, this was accompanied by intense anxiety and unease … I spent that New Year in extreme distress.
[这一住就是五个月. 开始是打冬眠针, 后来换吃氯氮平, 效果都不好, 最后采用胰岛素休克疗法, 治疗了四十多天, 病情才逐渐稳定, 但仍然残留了一部分幻听 … 我复学了, 但每天有十四五个小时都在昏睡中度过, 醒来后也无精打采的 … 由于长期服用氯氮平, 出院两年后, 我的血液白细胞数骤减, 只

好换药, 开始吃复康素. 当时我正准备回家过年, 医生说, 这次可以痊愈了, 我也很高兴. 可事实恰好相反, 我对复康素的反应十分强烈, 坐卧不宁, 幻听有大量出现了, 并且伴有强烈的焦虑、心慌 … 这个新年我是在极端的痛苦中度过的.]

(Text 6, Yao 2000, 331)

Explanatory models of mental illness

In seeking to make sense of an illness experience people will draw on 'explanatory models' consisting of 'beliefs about illness, the personal and social meaning of the illness, expectations about what will happen as a result of illness, how a healer is expected to intervene, and what therapeutic goals are held' (Cora-Bramble and Williams 2000, 265). These explanatory models embraced by individuals may have diverse origins: cultural, professional, institutional and political, amongst others. Moreover, an individual may embrace more than one explanatory model at any stage of his or her illness as well as change his or her preferred explanatory model over time (Bury 2001; Williams and Healy 2001). It is common in the case of mental illness, for example, that a biomedical (professional) explanatory model and a cultural explanatory model may be concurrently embraced (Callan and Littlewood 1998; Kleinman 1980; McCabe and Priebe 2004).

Despite the psychoeducational context of publication of the life stories under study, only three draw on the biomedical explanatory model when contemplating the aetiological basis of mental illness.

For instance, if I suddenly get the idea, in a paranoid delusion, that I suspect there is poison in my food, what do I do? This is how I think: if there really is poison then I will die on eating the food; if there is no poison and I retaliate against him [the believed perpetrator], it would mean that I have probably fallen ill again. Of these two, which do I choose? I choose to sooner die an unnatural death than to be willing to fall ill again. In fact, facing many more such things just proves over and over again that it is illness. What's more, when it reoccurs my mind remembers this and the abnormal neurons get transformed.
[例如我怀疑饭里有毒, 出现被害妄想一闪念, 怎么办? 我这么想, 要是真有毒我吃了死了, 要是没有毒我报复他很可能犯病. 这两条我选择哪条呢? 选择我宁可死于非命也不愿选择再犯病. 在事实面前这样的事多了, 多次证明它是病了, 再出现时脑子就长记性了, 异常的脑细胞就得到改造了.]

(Text 4, Yao 2000, 321)

Why did I join the special life circle of mental illness? This has a definite connection to my genes.
[我为什么进入精神病这个特殊的生活圈子, 这跟我的基因有一定关系.]

(Text 13, Yao 2000, 341–342)

My illness is hereditary. My grandma and my mother both developed mental illness at the age of 16.
[我的病是遗传的, 我的姥姥、母亲都在16岁时发过精神病。]

(Text 22, Yao 2007, 2)

These references to the biomedical explanatory model of mental illness locate the aetiological basis of mental illness in neuronal disorder and biogenetics. There is no reference to specific pathogenetic factors, such as neurotransmitter irregularities, in any of the stories. This occurs despite psychoeducational programs in mainland China typically detailing the pathophysiological basis to mental illness (Ran *et al.* 2003; Yang and Pearson 2002; Yip 2007)[9], in line with the paradigmatic dominance of the biomedical explanatory model in mainland Chinese psychiatry (Kleinman and Kleinman 1985; Pearson 1995a; Phillips 1993; Ran *et al.* 2005; Tseng 1986). In addition, this occurs despite the fact that all the authors of the stories are taking prescribed medications that regulate neurotransmitters.

Resonance of the biomedical explanatory model in the narrative corpus may be even lower when one considers that the hereditary potential of mental illness has long been recognised in Chinese tradition and contributes appreciably to the intense stigma toward mental illness observed in Chinese societies even today (Ramsay 2008). Thus, the two authors' references in Texts 13 and 22 above to a biogenetic aetiology could equally stem from the cultural explanatory model of mental illness informed by Chinese tradition.

The aetiological explanatory model most resonant in the stories, in fact, is the psychosocial model. Life stresses and pressures, more so than physiology and biology, are often recounted as important aetiological factors in mental illness.

At university, although there was no academic pressure, the cause of my disease – the pressure of social interaction – however, remained. Eventually, in 1995 I experienced auditory hallucinations and delusions and was diagnosed with early stage schizophrenia.
[在大学里, 虽然没有学习上的压力, 但我的病因 – 社交上的压力却依然存在, 终于1995年出现了幻听、妄想, 被诊断为精神分裂症前期。]

(Text 15, Yao 2000, 347–348)

Excessive academic pressure and not getting used to university life caused me to eventually fall ill. At hospital I was diagnosed as suffering from mental illness.
[过重的学习压力和对大学生活的不适应使我终于病倒了。我被医院诊断患了精神病。]

(Text 17, Yao 2000, 352)

Pearson (1995c, 1166) reports the salience of the psychosocial explanatory model of mental illness in cohorts of urban dwelling clients and family caregivers in mainland China, pointing out that '[t]his is not a frame of reference that Chinese doctors usually share.'

Finally, there is also evidence of individuals simultaneously embracing multiple explanatory models (Garro 2000). In the following example biomedical (and/or cultural), psychosocial and dietary explanations are concurrently proposed.

> The reason for me falling ill is, firstly, heredity: my father had a mental illness. Another factor is psychological upsets in adulthood, including being jilted in love and being unfairly criticised, amongst others. In addition, there is malnutrition from the difficult times, for example, and also my character is fairly introverted, having been classified as split personality. This is also a factor.
> [得病的原因一是遗传, 我父亲有精神病; 另一方面是后天的精神刺激, 包括失恋、不公正地被批判等等. 另外, 比如说困难时期吃不饱饭, 还有自己性格比较内向, 属于分裂人格, 这也是一方面.]

(Text 4, Yao 2000, 318)

Comprehensive understanding

In Chapter 1 it is noted that meaning is expressed in people's stories of illness experiences through the temporal and causal ordering of life events, through an asserting and refashioning of identities, and through language use. Culture is deemed to shape these processes. The ensuing analysis explores these narrative processes as manifest in the mainland Chinese life stories of mental illness. This is undertaken by reference to the distinguishing semantic and linguistic structural features explicated above.

Mental illness in the life stories under study constitutes a temporal juncture in the person's life, marking out an embodied life in health and a disembodied life in illness (Kleinman *et al.* 2011; Traphagan 2000). Mental illness thus comprises a 'biographical disruption' (Bury 1982, 169) whereby life following the onset of illness is characterised by loss, for example, in finances, self-worth and future certainty. This is in contrast to the fulfilling life seemingly lived before. At the same time, this life from before serves as motivation for a future life in recovery, where the person can once again usefully contribute to society. The normative life pathway and attendant social responsibilities in Chinese culture shape such a notion of recovery, which is defined, not by individual needs and achievements, but by prescriptions pertaining to social functionality and worth (Kleinman *et al.* 2011; Traphagan 2000).

This culturally shaped aspiration designates future selves as continuous with past selves. There is little celebration or anticipation of the fashioning of new selves through the illness experience (Bury 2001; Frank 1998; Hawkins 1999; Hydén 1997). Mental illness, thus, is positioned as a temporary interlude. During this interlude, selves become defined by their illness. The name of the person's illness, acquired through the biomedical intervention and psychoeducational intervention experienced in hospital as an in-patient, is commonly embraced and asserted. The psychoeducational context of the publication of the stories in question, clearly, provides some explanation for this. Yet, the normative life pathway and attendant social responsibilities in Chinese culture also likely shape this process. The claiming of an illness identity can provide some sanctuary from the acute disembodiment people with a mental illness experience, at least within the family environ (Hunt 2000). The losses and unusual behaviours characterising mental illness are particularly discredited in Confucian-heritage societies, where great value is placed on order, harmony and the fulfilment of culturally prescribed roles (Pearson 1996; Traphagan 2000). Allowances are likely to be made for an inability to meet familial and social expectations, at least by loved ones, if personal circumstances are framed in terms of being ill.

In the life stories under study, the claiming of an illness identity also appears to proceed from imaginings of a commonality in the illness experience (Kohrman 2005), which connects people with a mental illness to a community of fellow sufferers, even though they have likely not met in person. The language employed in the storytelling accomplishes this by reconstituting an individual's singular illness experience into a collective one. This fulfils the need for those with a mental illness in a collectivist culture such as Chinese, for engagement with and connectedness to others in society. This, in turn, provides the support, hope and motivation of the (imagined) group as the individual journeys toward recovery. As a consequence, the 'bearing of witness' in the life stories of mental illness under study both 'requires community' (the newsletter readership) *and* 'creates community' (a community of fellow suffers) (Charon 2006, 197. See also Miller *et al*. 2005, 298, for discussion of how stories can 'function to *build community*' (original emphasis).)

This cultural prioritising of social relationships and defining self through connections with others can also explain the language of praise and acclaim directed toward broader society in the life stories. Complimentary language is used by the people with a mental illness, despite the intense stigma toward mental illness which pervades Chinese societies.[10] A cultural need for connection with others in society appears to silence any criticism of the broader society. It would likely be problematic for the people with a mental illness to represent in overtly negative terms the very thing that they so fervently seek to return to. For most, 'returning to society' constitutes the primary goal in recovery.

With this in mind, the battle metaphor becomes particularly suited to reconciling the depth of the personal challenges and losses which are experienced by the person with a mental illness, with the cultural expectation that recovery entails returning to a fully productive role in society. Stark differences in levels of social functioning separate the former from the latter. All three elements that Hawkins (1999) claims are required for the effective expression of the battle metaphor in illness (see Chapter 1) are in evidence in the stories in question, namely, an identified enemy (mental illness); an alliance with the health professional (working 'hand-in-hand' with the psychiatrist and psychologist);[11] and the use of therapeutic weaponry (psychotropic medication). While the battle metaphor also characterises illness stories from other cultural settings (see Chapter 1), there is familiar historical and political resonance in its usage in the life stories under study. This reflects a mainland Chinese population well versed in the language of battle and struggle as a result of its common use in the political discourse of the revolutionary past and the present-day reform period (Ramsay 1997; Trevaskes 2007).

The culturally shaped notion of recovery and forms of identity recounted in the life stories do not empower or grant political voice to those with a mental illness (Couser 1997). The stories appear to be located in Brody's (2003, 141) 'first stage' of illness testimony, where 'the sick ... gather in a mini-community, such as a support group made up solely of those who have suffered from the same sort of disease.' Brody's (2003, 141) 'second' activist stage, where 'the mini-community as a group can engage the larger community with its testimony', often by means of 'political measures' and social agitation, is not in evidence. The life stories of mental illness do not call for social equality, mandate participation in pharmacotherapeutic decision-making, or actively promote political agenda. Chinese cultural norms of behaviour likely shape this, with public harmony being valued over dissent and lay people being expected to defer to those with specialist knowledge, such as medical professionals (Fan and Karnilowicz 2000; Kleinman 1980; Kung 2001; Pearson 1995c; Ramsay 2008). This is likely compounded in the context of mainland China, where the political environment also tends to curb public activism.

Chinese cultural deference to those with specialist knowledge is further evident in the form of the patient and health professional relationship recounted in the life stories under study. Professional direction is adhered to without question, in line with Kleinman's (1980, 264) observation that, in the Chinese medical encounter, the health professional's 'secret knowledge, somewhat higher social status, and emotional distance are signs of his therapeutic power and, therefore, are an essential part of the doctor-patient relationship.' The degree of compliance with health professional directives by the person with a mental illness is such that even when therapeutic outcomes do not meet those promised at the outset of medical treatment – with low medication efficacy, residual symptomatology and distressing side-effects characterising pharmacotherapy in the stories under study – a person's continuing adherence to and her or his belief in the fundamental value of the therapeutic regime are rarely brought into question.

What is more, the frequently recounted negative therapeutic experiences do not appear to have been deemed problematic by the editor of the psychoeducational volumes where the life stories are published. No attempt has seemingly been made to modify or remove such references. The implication is that, in the mind of the editor of the psychoeducational publications, it is inconceivable that the weight of biomedical advice could be undermined by the recounted tales of poor pharmacotherapeutic outcomes. People will dutifully comply with health professional directives regardless of outcome, as this is what cultural norms compel them to do. Brody (2003, 160) considers such submission to biomedicine, as displayed in the life stories under study, to be highly disempowering in that the person 'stops being in the world in too many important ways and enters the prison of his disease instead.' In the life stories in question, the person appears to become both imprisoned by the illness *and* confined to the custody of the health professional. Such confinement is likely to be, at once, both disempowering and reassuring for the person with a mental illness, given that this is how Chinese cultural norms prescribe that the patient and health professional relationship should be.

Causal relationships documented in illness stories are particularly important in that they can reveal the salient explanatory models drawn on by people to make sense of their illness experience. In the stories under study there is minimal voicing of a biomedical aetiological explanation of mental illness. This occurs despite the psychoeducational context of publication of the stories and the documented hegemony of the biomedical explanatory model of mental illness in mainland Chinese mental health circles (Kleinman and Kleinman 1985; Pearson 1995a; Phillips 1993; Ran *et al.* 2005; Tseng 1986). Culture-based stigma likely shapes an observed preference for psychosocial aetiological explanations in the life stories. There is intense stigma against mental illness in Chinese culture, more so than that experienced in Western settings (Bahl 1999; Bentelspacher *et al.* 1994; Fan and Karnilowicz 2000; Loo *et al.* 1989; Phillips 1993; Ramsay 2008; Ran *et al.* 2005; Yang 2007). Goffman (quoted in Link *et al.* 2004, 512) defines stigma as 'an "attribute that is deeply discrediting" and that reduces the bearer "from a whole and usual person to a tainted, discounted one"'. The aforementioned disembodiment that attends mental illness, leaving the person unable to fulfil culturally prescribed roles, is one factor contributing to the stigma against people with a mental illness in Chinese culture (Kleinman *et al.* 2011; Yang and Kleinman 2008). Pearson (1996, 438) also notes the role of cultural norms of behaviour:

> Of all conditions, mental illness is one that confounds a culture that values conformity, discretion, modesty, and rectitude. The potential for disorder and nonconformity that severe mental disorder represents – particularly the symptoms of mania and schizophrenia – is deeply disturbing within Chinese society. Stigma and rejection of the mentally ill are common experiences in most societies, but in China they seem to be felt with a particular intensity.

Stigma against mental illness in Chinese culture is particularly intense as the perceived deficits and undesirable behaviours are seen to characterise a condition whose hereditary potential is long recognised in Chinese culture (Dikötter 1998; Lin 1981; Ramsay 2008; Ran *et al.* 2005). This makes the biomedical explanatory model of mental illness potentially problematic for lay Chinese, since the biomedical aetiological explanation for illnesses like schizophrenia points to genetic factors. Such an explanation, therefore, can readily be seen to legitimise the cultural stigma rooted in heredity (Ramsay 2008). Carabas and Harter (2005, 151) state that '[s]hame, embarrassment, and distrust evolve through the process of *othering* that stigmatization performs, and are embodied in people's life narratives.' In the life stories under study this manifests in a form of silencing (Beck *et al.* 2005; Harter *et al.* 2005; Kirmayer 2000; Riessman 1993; Squire 2005), with the people with a mental illness either being mindful not to openly embrace or choosing to reject the biomedical explanation for the cause of their illness, elements of which reinforce the culture-based stigma that they are very well aware of and would seek to avoid. Thus, a problematic intersection of biomedicine and culture may lead people to turn to a culturally more 'palatable' aetiological explanation in the stories in question, namely, a psychosocial explanation. There appears to be much less cultural shame attending an admission of succumbing to life's pressures as compared to exposing that one's family has tainted genes.

Equally, cultural stigma may explain the absence of reference to spiritual causes of mental illness in the life stories. This occurs despite the widespread belief, at least in rural China, that mental illness is caused by 'disturbances in the spirit world' (Li and Phillips 1990, 221. See also Yip 2007). It is noted at the outset of the current chapter that the people in the stories under study are unlikely to be from the peasant class. Nevertheless, some may be from small rural towns.[12] Any admission of spiritual possession would bring shame to these people and their families (Yip 2007), and, as a consequence, would silence the expression of a spiritual aetiology. Preference would be given to the culturally more palatable psychosocial aetiological explanation, as pointed out above.

Conclusion

Analysis of the mainland Chinese life stories of mental illness has found that culture and biomedicine often appear to 'collude' in ways that shape the stories in similar directions. Cultural expectations in recovery entail returning to a productive role in society, as was the case before mental illness intervened. Biomedicine provides the means by which this can be achieved, namely, pharmacotherapy (Ng *et al.* 2008a, 2008b, 2011). Cultural norms prescribe acquiescence to professional authority and direction (Kleinman 1980; Ramsay 2008). Biomedicine valorises medication compliance (Lam *et al.* 2011; Ng *et al.* 2008a). Cultural values motivate the claiming of an illness identity, where connection with others in a form of community can be fashioned and drawn on for support and motivation during the illness experience. The claiming of an illness identity may also partially assuage the cultural shame that stems from the disembodiment experienced in mental illness. Biomedicine names this illness identity.

This apparent complementarity in how culture and biomedicine shape the stories in question, of course, may not be coincidental. The people telling the stories have had some form of contact with formal mental health services, in contrast to the vast majority of people with a mental illness in mainland China, who remain untreated (Lee and Kleinman 2007; Pearson 1996; Ran *et al.* 2005). They have also likely read the stories that have preceded theirs, published in the psychoeducational newsletter forum. These experiences may have influenced their storytelling in ways that advance the biomedical agenda yet, at the same time, retain cultural connectedness. Frank (2009, 170) cautions that such collusion can be 'an especially prevalent danger in contemporary health care' in the West, where 'storytelling can be hijacked – appropriated and regulated – by institutional interests that want particular stories told in circumscribed ways, in order to advance a specific agenda.' This can produce life stories that are 'prepackaged' in ways that speak to cultural norms and prescriptions (Brody 2003, 159).

Whether the apparent complementarity between culture and biomedicine in the stories under study is calculated or subliminal, it is not absolute in expression. Culture, in the end, shapes selective engagement of the biomedical explanatory model of mental illness. The illness identity may be embraced and directives by health professionals rigorously adhered to, yet psychosocial rather than biological factors more commonly provide the aetiological explanation for mental illness in the stories in question. This occurs even though mental health professionals and public health bodies in mainland China tend to promote the latter over the former (Pearson 1995a, 1995c). In so doing, the storytellers are looking to an explanatory model of mental illness that does not call to mind cultural stigma rooted in heredity.

In sum, the life stories analysed in this chapter are culturally shaped in ways that likely provide a sense of comfort to the storyteller. A degree of certainty and continuity is offered in the people's disrupted lives with a promise of recovery and a return to society. The heroic efforts required to achieve this are reconciled through culturally familiar metaphors of struggle and battle. At the same time, the self from before illness is restored in the imaginings of the future self. Moreover, solace is found in the illness community and in social support and by engaging an aetiological explanation that moderates the potential shame brought to the individual and family.

The price of this comfort is disempowerment. A sense of future new selves do not emerge in the stories told (Bury 2001; Frank 1998; Hawkins 1999; Hydén 1997). More value is placed on the restitution of the old self. Recovery is culturally ascribed rather than individually negotiated based on personal wishes and goals (Ng *et al.* 2011, 2012), even though holding down a job, being productive in the workforce, and meeting the norms of social interaction remain problematic in mental illness. Life circumstances are rarely contested or agitated against and medication compliance is adhered to despite the frequently less than optimal outcomes recounted. What emerge are life stories where cultural understandings, norms, values and scripts, at once, alleviate and add to the burden of the experience of mental illness for the person with a mental illness.

3 Life stories of family caregiving in mental illness

In Chapter 2 we explored how culture shapes life stories written by mainland Chinese people with a mental illness. In this chapter we examine how culture shapes life stories written by mainland Chinese people caring for a family member with mental illness. Examination of the stories of family caregivers is believed to be particularly important in the context of mental illness in mainland China, given that over 90 per cent of people with schizophrenia, for instance, live at home with their families (Phillips 1993; Ran *et al*. 2005; Yip 2007). This is corroborated in the personal corpus analysed in Chapter 2 where the stories of adult-children residing in the family home dominate.

The family caregiver stories under study in the current chapter were located in the same edited volumes from where the personal stories analysed in Chapter 2 were sourced. Once again, the family caregiver stories had originally been published in a 'letters to the editor' style of format in the monthly psychoeducational newsletter, *Mental Illness Recovery News*. Life stories and other material from the newsletter had been selected for inclusion in the volumes by the editor, Professor Yao Guizhong. As in Chapter 2, the family caregiver stories from the two edited volumes were eventually combined and analysed together as a single 'family caregiver' corpus composed of 29 life stories. The stories range from approximately 400 to 2000 characters in length (approximating 300 to 1500 English words) and speak of family caregiving in severe mental illness, including schizophrenia and clinical depression, as follows:

- eighteen schizophrenia stories;
- two clinical depression stories;
- nine 'mental illness' (diagnostic name unspecified) stories.

The vast majority of the nine stories that did not specify a diagnostic name for the mental illness in question speak of psychotic experiences in their narrative content. Experiences of schizophrenia/psychotic illness, therefore, dominate the family caregiver corpus as they did the personal corpus analysed in Chapter 2.

Nineteen authors were identifiable as women (eighteen mothers and one daughter), four as men (three fathers and one husband), with the remaining six of undeterminable gender (five parents and one undetermined kinship). It is likely that at least half of the five parents of undeterminable gender are mothers, leaving the family caregiver corpus dominated by the stories of mothers as primary caregivers. A gender imbalance toward women in caregiving in illness, particularly mothers, is documented in the existing research, which finds that this is particularly the case in Confucian-heritage societies such as mainland China (Brown and Alligood 2004; Harden 2005; Holroyd and Mackenzie 1995; Lin and Lu 2005; Milliken 2001; Pearson and Tsang 2004; Pierret 2003; Stern *et al.* 1999; Wong *et al.* 2004; Yip 2007; Yu and Chau 1997). Holroyd (2001, 1127) states that these 'intimate and feminine aspects of caring are not so much the result of the sexual division of labour within the family as they are the organizing principle around which this division is built.' Overall, the fact that all bar three authors in the family caregiver corpus are parents reflects the typical age of onset of the illnesses in question, usually late teens or twenties, and the difficulty of marrying off family members with a mental illness in mainland China (Phillips 1993).

The socioeconomic status and class backgrounds of the family caregivers match those of the people with a mental illness who authored the counterpart stories analysed in Chapter 2. The limitations and benefits of using the public stories under study as sources of data also accord with those described in Chapter 2.

Analysis of family caregiver life stories of mental illness[1]

This chapter follows the analytic procedure laid out in Chapter 2 in explicating how culture shapes the mainland Chinese life stories of family caregiving in mental illness.

Naïve understanding

Taken together, the life stories under study portray mental illness as a catastrophic event for the families concerned, who face many hurdles in their struggle to provide care to their ill family members. As with the personal stories, loss is salient to the experience of mental illness, including financial loss, future uncertainty for caregiver and ill family member alike, and, particularly where violence is experienced, loss of family cohesion and stability. Through at times protracted and convoluted pathways to medical care, the family caregiver, mostly mother or wife, responds with exhaustive efforts to have the family member treated and 'cured'. Doing anything less brings certain shame and guilt. The primary goal of the family is to assist and guide the ill family member toward 'recovery', thereby ensuring that they are able to play a fully productive and contributory role in society. Family caregivers are also fully aware of the acute shame in having a family member with mental illness, so efforts are made to ensure that people beyond the family unit are not aware of and are unable to ascertain the ill family member's diagnosis. Family caregivers are expected to and, for the most part, are willing to exert all necessary effort to effect these goals, no matter the sacrifices required and the demands or burdens this places on the caregiver and the healthy family members. In maintaining a high level of commitment to their role, family caregivers reveal a prevailing sense of hope and positivity toward the existing circumstances and the future of the ill family member, although this rarely extends to the caregiver personally, for example, through developing a sense of personal achievement and valuing attendant gains in self-efficacy. Reflecting the psychoeducational context of publication of the stories, regular contact with mental health services and compliance with professionally prescribed pharmacotherapeutic regimes are presented as caregiver responsibilities and essential facets to the ill family member's recovery. Directions by medical professionals are dutifully respected and adhered to by family caregivers, even though pharmacotherapeutic outcomes often do not meet that promised or expected at the outset of treatment.

Sentence level structural analysis

Analysis of the sentence level linguistic and semantic features of the life stories under study reveals the following salient themes and subthemes pertaining to the family caregiver experience of mental illness (Table 3.1). They are discussed and illustrated subsequently.

Mental illness is a family tragedy

The family is the fundamental unit in Chinese society (Yip 2007). According to Confucian teachings, social harmony is contingent on intra-familial harmony. Harmony is maintained when family members are respectful of and are able to carry out their 'prescribed roles' and duties (Braun and Browne 1998, 264). It is important that the projected life pathways of family members are realised so that reciprocal responsibilities to one another can be fulfilled. Any disruption of this has significant ramifications not only for the family concerned but for the wider society.

In the life stories under study, deeply negative and intense language is frequently employed by caregivers to describe the tragic impact of mental illness on the family. While studies of Western life stories also feature the dramatic changes that mental illness brings to afflicted individuals and their families (Bengs *et al.* 2008; Hayne and Yonge 1997; Jones 2005; Wisdom *et al.* 2008), the mainland Chinese caregiver stories are commonly marked by a particularly 'extreme' lexicon and a focus as much on the familial repercussions as on the impact on the ill individual per se. These repercussions are characteristically narrated figuratively, heavily drawing on the material metaphor of natural disaster to describe the experience rather than direct reference to personal emotion. Hydén (1995, 73) observes that such use of figurative language in life stories of mental illness told in the West serves as a 'way of recategorizing events and actions, of "customizing" disruptive phenomena that were initially alien ... by incorporating them into [the] everyday world.'

Table 3.1 Salient themes and subthemes in mainland Chinese family caregiver stories of mental illness

Theme	Subtheme
Mental illness is a family tragedy	Mental illness is catastrophic
	Protracted pathway to diagnosis
	Mental illness is a battle
	Episodes of violence
Mental illness causes loss	Financial cost of mental illness
	Loss of future expectations
	Family instability
Obligation to care	Caregiving is a familial responsibility
	Caregiving 'at any cost'
	Self-blame and guilt
	Desire to escape from caregiving responsibility
Maintenance of hope and positivity	Value of hope and positivity
Role of society in 'recovery' of the ill family member	'Returning' to society
	Social stigma and concealment
Biomedical intervention	Non-compliance leads to relapse
	Pharmacotherapeutic failure, residual symptomatology and medication side-effects
Explanatory models of mental illness	Mental illness has a biomedical aetiology
	Mental illness has a psychosocial aetiology

My child, to whom I had given a lifetime of painstaking care to raise to adulthood, developed a mental illness. My life in its later years had become dark and desolate. My family was torn to pieces. I felt waves of heartfelt pain and was in an indefinite state of panic. I unremittingly sensed the approach of a great earthquake.

[我的孩子, 我付出毕生心血抚养大的孩子得了精神病. 我的晚年生活变得灰暗凄凉, 我的家变得支离破碎. 我阵阵心痛, 惊魂不定, 时时预感到大地震的降临].

(Text II, Yao 2000, 246)

My husband and I were with him day and night and felt that what our son spoke about was a bit strange, so we managed to take him to a hospital mental health unit to seek medical advice. The doctor diagnosed that he was suffering from schizophrenia. At the time it was like being struck by lightning five times in succession. There is simply no way to express the despondency and dismay we felt in our hearts.

[我和老伴与他朝夕相处, 觉得他讲话的内容有些异常, 就设法送他到一家医院精神科就诊. 医师诊断他患的是精神分裂症. 当时我们如同五雷击顶, 其内心的失望和惊恐简直无法言表].

(Text VII, Yao 2000, 262)

A notable feature of the tragedy for many family caregivers is the protracted and tortuous pathways that are often negotiated before obtaining the diagnosis of mental illness and receiving appropriate treatment for the family member's condition. Delayed presentation of Chinese people with a mental illness to health authorities has been well documented in the clinical research (Wong 2000; Wong *et al.* 2003; Yang and Kleinman 2008).[2] In the life stories under study, many family caregivers often at first attribute the observed symptoms to behaviours arising from everyday pressures or the stresses of modern life in mainland China and seek to keep the matter in-house. For some, intra-familial conflict arises over the aetiology of the observed symptoms, with refusal by some family members to contemplate a biomedical origin. Where help is sought outside the family, Chinese folk therapies usually constitute the first port of call, including traditional Chinese medicine and spiritual healing (Li and Phillips 1990). When formal health services are eventually sought out, first contact often involves misdiagnosis, leading to greater delay in the reaching of a correct diagnosis and caregiver disenchantment and disappointment with these services.

At that time, my home was a constant scene of war; the smell of gunpowder permeated everywhere. Looking back now, these were early signs of my son's developing illness, but at the time who would have known! All the time I thought it was just my child growing up, refusing to accept discipline …. I took him to the hospital for an examination and the doctor said that these were signs of neurasthenia[3] and sent him back to school with some Oryzanol and sedatives. His condition did not gradually improve but only grew worse …. I took him to several hospitals who all thought he had neurasthenia …. In early 1996, despite family objections (my mother-in-law is superstitious and thought it was 'Deficiency of Qi' and so made her grandson also seek a cure from the 'gods'), I single-mindedly took my child to Anding Hospital in Beijing[4] …. He had two consecutive stays in Anding Hospital lasting for over ten months and yet still no clear-cut diagnosis: what was I to do?

[那个时期, 我家里战火频频, 到处充满了火药味. 现在回忆起来, 这就是我儿子得病的早期表现, 那时候谁知道哇! 我总认为, 这是孩子长大了, 不服管教了 … 我带他去医院检查, 大夫说, 这是神经衰弱的表现, 带了点儿谷维素、安定等药, 就回校上课去了. 病情并没有逐渐缓解, 而是向深处发展 … 我带他跑了几家医院, 都认为他是神经衰弱 … 1996年初, 我不顾家人的反对 (婆婆迷信, 认为这是"虚症", 让孙子也求治于"神灵") 毅然带着孩子到了北京安定医院 … 在安定医院, 先后住了两次院, 历时10个多月, 还没有一个明确的诊断, 我该怎么办呢?]

(Text V, Yao 2000, 254–255)

I was also very much shocked by the sudden changes in my son and would cry out, in turn, 'what's going on here?' Even so, I still took my son's various anomalies to be part of the 'one-child phenomenon' that people nowadays are very familiar with. I mistakenly took the mental illness he was suffering from to be a psychological impediment and personality defect shaped by the affluence of the modern family and mollycoddling by parents. Furthermore, I had no way of knowing that my son's cognitive reversal was in fact a manifestation of early stage schizophrenia.

Thus, in subsequent treatment, although we loved our child very much and were extremely anxious for him to get treatment, in the end we didn't understand the main issue. We aimlessly sought medical treatment. As a result, only the superficial symptoms were treated instead of the root cause of his illness .... Unfortunately, we lacked confidence in the treatment methods of specialist hospitals, rather believing, as people say in the community, that 'one must rely on traditional Chinese medicine to treat illness' .... Fortunately, we eventually opted to go to a regular hospital for in-patient treatment and from thereon began to obtain a proper diagnosis and treatment.

[儿子突如其来的变化也令我震惊不已, 连呼这是怎么了? 即使这样, 我还是把儿子种种异常当成当代人都耳熟目睹的"独生子女现象", 把儿子患有的精神疾病错当成现代家庭条件优裕、父母溺爱娇惯形成的心理障碍和人格缺陷, 更无从得知儿子认知逆转即是精神分裂症的早期现象。

所以在此后的治疗中, 虽然我们疼孩子心切, 急如星火, 但终因不得要领, 盲目投医, 往往舍本治表, 没治到病根上 ... 可惜我们对专科医院的治疗手段缺乏信任, 转而相信了社会上传说的"治病还得靠中医" ... 庆幸的是我们终于选择了到正规医院住院治疗, 并由此开始得到了正确的诊治。]

(Text XII, Yao 2000, 276–278)

Like the personal stories analysed in Chapter 2, in facing the tragedy that mental illness brings to families and in negotiating the protracted pathways to correct diagnosis and treatment, the battle metaphor is commonly drawn on in the family caregiver stories. In so doing, the family caregivers frequently refer to (biomedical) knowledge as an essential weapon in the battle against mental illness. Once again, the language used by family caregivers possesses clear historical and political resonance, locating their effort within a wider system of sociocultural meaning and reference (Kleinman 1988) that embodies the invested effort as 'heroic' (Bury 2001; Carney 2004).

When he was capable of listening I would pick out a section to read to him so as to make him understand his condition and be able to properly triumph over it .... In a word, he began to correct his bad habits and knew to wage a struggle against his illness (laziness and withdrawal).

[在他能听时, 我就选择一段读给他听, 让他明白自己的病情, 好战胜它 ... 总之他开始改正自己的坏习惯了, 懂得同疾病 (懒散退缩) 作斗争了].

(Text XV, Yao 2000, 285–286)

To date my child retains some residual symptoms, such as passiveness and laziness, and cannot undertake regular work or study. Take your time and do not worry about these symptoms that won't change for a period of time. You must be mentally prepared to fight a protracted battle.
[我的孩子至今还残留着某些症状, 比如: 被动、懒散, 不能正常工作或学习, 对这些一时还改变不了的症状, 不能着急, 慢慢来, 要有打持久战的思想准备.]

(Text XIX, Yao 2000, 300)

As a parent, firstly, my spirit must never fail; secondly, I must increase my knowledge and, having acquired the weapons, only then can I help the ill person triumph over his or her disease.
[我作为家长, 一是精神不能倒, 二是要加强学习, 掌握了武器才能帮助病人战胜疾病.]

(Text XXIII, Yao 2007, 91)

For some, the heavy burden of facing the tragedy of mental illness or the protracted pathway to correct diagnosis and treatment of the family member with a mental illness leads to episodes of violence. While not dominant across the corpus, more than one-quarter of the stories under study, nevertheless, speak of violence in the family environs. This represents a fairly high incidence, given that only 'a modest association' has been found 'between major mental illness and violence' (Hiday 1995, 122. See also Glick and Applbaum, 2010, and Kleinman *et al.*, 2011). Hiday (1995, 123) cites research which confirms 'that most mentally ill people were not violent; only a small minority with major mental illness (7%) committed any violent acts in the previous year.'

The recounting of violence in the family caregiver corpus well exceeds that of the personal corpus. Moreover, the recounted violence manifests both in the actions of the person with a mental illness, mostly exhibited during the lengthy period before obtaining a correct diagnosis and treatment, as well as in the actions of the family caregiver, for the most part arising from frustration with the disembodiment attending mental illness (see Chapter 2, and Kleinman *et al.* 2011).

My son had not yet reached one month of age when he suffered quite a few beatings because of crying noisily at night and disturbing his [mentally ill father's] sleep. He [the father] was unable to accept it and got terribly angry over what, for ordinary people, would seem very petty things … He paid no attention at all to our son's study and his life, and regularly came to blows over some very trivial matters …. His father's violent behaviour was commonplace to him.
[儿子出生没过满月, 就因为晚上哭闹吵了他的觉挨了好几次打. 在常人看来很小的事, 他却无法接受而大发脾气 ... 儿子的学习、生活他全然不管, 为点鸡毛蒜皮的事儿, 经常大打出手 ... 他父亲的粗暴行为是他司空见惯了.]

(Text V, Yao 2000, 253–254)

Because she didn't have a job, she was in an unhappy frame of mind, dispirited and downcast all day long. She just ate and slept. She just lazed about all day long, not wanting to do anything. We often vented our feelings about this and constantly argued. I even beat and abused her, saying she was a disappointment and a good-for-nothing. I even didn't give her food to eat to force her to get a job.

[由于没有工作, 心情不舒畅, 整天无精打采, 除了吃饭就是睡, 整天懒得要命, 什么也不想干, 为此我们没少闹矛盾, 经常吵架, 我甚至打她、骂她, 说她不争气, 没出息, 甚至不给她饭吃, 逼她去工作.]

(Text XIV, Yao 2000, 280)

Mental illness causes loss

The losses family caregivers recount focus on the financial costs and burdens, and future uncertainty. Both of these featured in the personal life stories and have been found to be salient to the family caregiving experience in the West (Harden 2005; Milliken 2001; Öhman and Söderberg 2004; Stern *et al.* 1999; Tuck *et al.* 1997). In the mainland Chinese family caregiver stories, the drain on family finances is quite onerous, leaving many living a subsistence mode of existence. As noted earlier, mainland Chinese families now face a user-pays health care system arising out of the post-1978 market-style economic reform program (Kohrman 2005; Yip 2007), yet many lack adequate medical insurance coverage (Pearson and Lam 2002). This is particularly problematic for parent caregivers approaching retirement age, who had expectations of economic security and reasonable comfort in this later period of their lives. Urban dwellers who had worked for state-owned industries and the government would also remember the free or heavily subsidised health care that they had enjoyed before the reform program. Financial uncertainty, in turn, contributes to the sense of future uncertainty expressed in the life stories, once again particularly for elder caregivers.

At the time I really felt that the end of the world was approaching. She [the wife] did not have medical insurance and, of course, no workplace would cough up for such expenses. We were extremely hard pressed for money. On top of the rent there was not much to put aside. We also spent a fair bit on our trip to Qingdao. There was now very little remaining.

There was no choice but to borrow money from anywhere we could. I was limited in what I could do, and there were no relatives in Beijing, just a few friends and neighbours who also didn't have much money. We could only afford treatment as an out-patient.

[我当时很有些世界末日来临的感觉. 她没有公费医疗, 当然没有单位来出这笔钱, 我们的手中也甚为拮据, 除了租房, 也没有多少积蓄, 去青岛又花了不少, 现在已所剩无几了.

没有办法, 只能四处去借钱. 我的活动能力有限, 北京又没有亲戚, 仅有的几个朋友或邻居, 也没有那么多钱, 只能在门诊治疗了.]

(Text IX, Yao 2000, 270)

My daughter had only been working for a year and did not have medical insurance. Over the past ten or so years she has been admitted to hospital three times, costing a lot of money. All the family savings have been spent on her visits to the doctor. We have spent a total of 2563 Yuan[5] 2 Jiao[6] in the six months since changing to Risperdal, needing to spend on average 427 Yuan 2 Jiao on medication each month. My daughter gets 494 Yuan salary each month and gives me 200 Yuan for living expenses. The remaining money is insufficient to cover medication, so each month I still need to subsidise her medication costs by 200 or so Yuan. My husband and I have been retired for 11 years. We have illnesses of our own and also need to visit the doctor and take medication. There is very little money left over each month. I worry about who would wish to be lumbered with her medical expenses once we pass away?

[我女儿刚参加工作一年, 没有公费医疗, 十多年来, 住了三次院, 花了不少钱, 家里的积蓄都给他看病了. 自从改服维思通以来, 6个月共花了2563.2元, 平均一个月得花药费427.20元. 我女儿每月工资494元, 给我生活费200元, 剩下钱吃药都不够, 我每月还得贴她药费200多元. 我和老伴已退休11年, 我们自己也有病, 也得看病吃药, 每月的钱所剩无几. 我担心一旦我们去世, 谁来负担她的医药费?]

(Text XIV, Yao 2000, 282–283)

Mental illness can also weaken family member bonds, of particular concern in family-centred societies such as mainland China. Specifically where violence in the home is encountered in the life stories under study, caregivers lament the damage this inflicts on the cohesion and integrity of the family unit.

Although I have a family of four, sometimes it's four people in four different places. When we want to speak to each other, we have to agree to meet somewhere in the street. And since we are all in a poor frame of mind, we speak then part on bad terms and, once again, go our separate ways.

[我虽是四口之家, 但有时是四个人在四个地方, 有话想说时, 只好相约在街头, 由于心情都不好, 谈的不欢而散, 就又各奔东西了.]

(Text II, Yao 2000, 247)

Your father and I are leaving this 'home'; we'll each find our own place to stay. He wants to go to a retirement home; I have also long decided to go to a retirement home for my remaining years. We, forever, will never again have a 'home'.

[我和你爸爸离开这个"家", 各找各的归宿. 他想去养老院, 我也早已决定去养老院了此余生, 咱们永远不会再有"家"了.]

(Text XVI, Yao 2000, 287)

Obligation to care

The familial obligation to care is extremely potent across the family caregiver corpus. This has been well documented in the clinical research (Pearson and

Lam 2002; Pearson and Ning 1997; Pearson and Tsang 2004; Phillips 1993; Yang and Pearson 2002). In the life stories under study this obligation to care for a family member with mental illness is never questioned or subject to qualification, despite the substantial losses that accompany the experience.

For the most part the responsibility to give care is carried out warmly and supportively, culturally consistent with the caregiver's role as parent to the person with a mental illness (caregivers being parents in all bar three stories). There are also clear didactic and interventionist elements to this care, with caregivers commonly 'guiding' [引导, 指导], 'supervising' [督促, 监控] and 'training' [训练, 疏导] the ill family member in life matters. They also ensure that the family member complies with pharmacotherapeutic regimes and maintains cooperation with the health professional. There is scant reference to the fostering of independence in decision-making, life autonomy and self-reliance in the family member with mental illness. Moreover, when permitted, this commonly leads to illness relapse and failure.

> I know from personal experience that it is extremely important for families to offer genuine, selfless love to restore the injured mind of the sufferer and to actively create a relaxed environment with family harmony, mutual respect and equal affection filled with human warmth. We must spare no effort in making the sufferer feel warm and happy in aspects of his or her life, mind and finances, amongst others …. I … need to encourage him to develop his interest (photography) and to create opportunities for social activities. In particular, I need to watch over his inner manoeuvrings and vexations, and become a person he can rely on and trust.
> [以我亲身体会, 家属用真挚无私的爱心来修复患者受伤的心灵, 积极创造一个家庭和睦、互相尊重、平等友爱、充满人间温暖的宽松环境是至关重要的. 要尽力让患者在生活、精神、经济等方面感受到愉快和温馨 … 我 … 要鼓励他发展自己的爱好 (摄影), 创造社交活动的机会, 尤其要观察他的内心活动与烦恼, 成为他可依靠和信赖的人.]
>
> (Text III, Yao 2000, 250)

> Although this task is difficult, who made me her mother? I have a responsibility to complete this arduous duty; this is also the aspiration of the families of every sufferer. Step-by-step we must climb up out of the deep abyss that is this serious illness. Only this way can we see the light and our child or loved one be saved.
> [虽然这项工作很艰苦, 但是谁让我是她的母亲呢? 我有责任完成这项艰巨的任务, 这也是我们每一位患者家属的心声, 我们一定要从这病魔的万丈深渊里一步一步地爬上来, 这样才能见到光明, 我们的孩子或亲人才能得救.]
>
> (Text XVIII, Yao 2000, 294)

> Thereupon, we no longer followed after him to watch over and protect him. We let him take his medication himself. For the first few weeks he was able to take a dose every now and then. Then for six months or more

he basically didn't take any medication .... In early April 2003, his workplace notified home, saying that lately his situation had not been good: he was not concentrating his efforts and his line of thought was confused .... Many years of watching over and protecting him had been destroyed in an instant.

[于是, 我们不再跟着陪护, 让他自己服药. 开始几周, 他还能隔三差五地服一次, 后来的半年多, 他基本上没有服药 ... 2003年4月初, 单位通知家里, 说他近来情况不好, 精力不集中, 思维混乱 ... 多年的陪护毁于一旦.]

(Text XXVI, Yao 2007, 98)

In many of the life stories under study, the caregiving responsibility is fully carried out regardless of the cost to the caregiver or, at times, her or his family. Caregivers direct all their efforts toward 'rescuing' [救] the family member with a mental illness, even to the detriment of spousal relations, relations with healthy siblings, or the caregiver's own life. All sacrifices are endured, with family caregiving viewed as a long-term endeavour.

We ... must not hesitate to do everything to cure our child's illness ... and to provide her with all the necessary conditions ... We look after her, understand her, respect her, don't impose on her and actively guide her, enabling her to have full confidence in life.

We have done everything for the sake of our child's recovery.

[我们 ... 要不惜一切把孩子的病治好 ... 并为她提供一切必要的条件 ... 我们关心她、理解她、尊重她, 不强加于她, 又积极引导她, 使她对生活充满信心.

我们为孩子的康复付出了一切.]

(Text X, Yao 2000, 271–272)

My relationship with his father was not good. I devoted all my love to my [ill] son .... I madly took my son to see doctors all over the place, disregarding my exhaustion, the cold and hunger.

[我与他爸感情不好, 我把所有的爱都倾注在儿子身上了 ... 我疯了似的到处给孩子看病, 不知疲倦, 不知冷, 也不知饿.]

(Text XIX, Yao 2000, 298)

Failure to fulfil the obligation to give appropriate care is a source of guilt for the family caregivers. Self-blame arises where caregivers see themselves as having failed to recognise the early signs of mental illness, in the knowledge that early treatment leads to better prognoses in mental illness; where caregivers see themselves as having contributed to a protracted pathway to correct diagnosis and treatment, due to misreading of symptoms or prioritising folk remedies and traditional Chinese medicine early on; and where parent caregivers see their long-term, committed efforts failing to stabilise their child's mental illness, attributing this failure wholly to their bad parenting skills: 'I am an incompetent mother' [我是一个不称职的母亲] (Text V, Yao 2000, 256).

Indeed, in the life stories under study self-blame for mental illness developing in a family member or for deemed poor outcomes in recovery is much more resonant than blame squarely directed at the illness itself (biomedical explanatory model) or blame attributed to actions of the ill family member.

> So, why have we spent all the time since our son fell ill relentlessly seeking a cure, yet in the end it turns out just the opposite? We have turned this over in our minds again and again, only to have the feeling that this is all on account of our ignorance …. Have we not paid a small price? Can we still make up for the difficulty that our time-wasting and procrastination have created for treatment? As soon as I think of these things I feel uneasy.
> [那么，为什么儿子得病以来我们一直求治不辍，最后却适得其反呢？我们反思再三，才感到这都是因为我们无知造成的 … 我们付出的代价还少吗？因为耽误、迁延而给治疗造成的困难还能弥补吗？一想到这些，我便惴惴不安。]
>
> (Text XII, Yao 2000, 275, 278)

> I am the one who has sinned … On reflection, why hasn't my child seen any improvement over time? One reason is the delay in treatment; another reason is that my vile moods have had a negative impact, causing my child to feel that he has an incurable disease: otherwise, why would Mummy be so scared?
> [一切罪过都归我 … 我回忆，为什么孩子迟迟不见好转？一方面是治疗不及时，再一方面是我的恶劣情绪起了负效应，使孩子感到自己得了不治之症. 要不，为什么妈妈吓成这样呢？]
>
> (Text XIX, Yao 2000, 298–299)

> It is definitely my fault that my child got sick …. As early as six months previously my son had signs of illness – such as anxiety, insomnia and keeping to himself. By the onset of illness on 19 August 2001, there was a process of quantitative to qualitative change. However, my love for my child was not properly expressed. All that I displayed was a harshness, rigidity and sobriety.
> [孩子病了肯定是我的过失 … 早在半年前，儿子就有了得病的征兆 — 心烦、失眠、独来独往等. 到2001年8月19号发病，这之中有个量变到质变的过程. 而我对孩子的爱并没有正确表现出来，表现出的只有严厉、严格、严肃.]
>
> (Text XXVIII, Yao 2007, 106–107)

Rarely do family caregivers express a desire to escape from caregiving responsibilities. Where this is expressed, the burden of caregiving at any cost has commonly been magnified by episodes of violence in the home. Escaping from caregiving duties entails physical distancing, by the caregiver leaving the home and, thus, the family member with mental illness; or by hospitalising the ill family member.

Because home life was turbulent, I stayed with others all over the place. I spent a couple of nights here then a couple of nights there …. Later on, I could not stay at home during the daytime and so would roam the streets.
[由于家里不安宁, 我到处借宿, 东家呆两天, 西家住两天 … 以后白天我不能在家呆, 就在街上逛。]

(Text II, Yao 2000, 247)

I did not know what I had done wrong. I experienced this kind of thing many times when Dad fell ill and really felt quite hurt. I could only relax a little when Dad was in hospital.
[不知道自己做错了什么?   这样的事情在爸爸患病期间我还遇到过很多次, 确实感到很委屈, 我只有在爸爸住院的时候才感到轻松一些。]

(Text IV, Yao 2000, 252)

When I was young I also thought of divorce. But due to remnants of feudal ethics and for the sake of my child, in the end I did not leave [my ill husband].
[年轻时也想到过离婚, 由于封建礼教的残余, 也为了孩子, 终究没有离成。]

(Text V, Yao 2000, 254)

Two mothers contemplate taking their own lives together with those of their children with mental illness. This may be attributable as much to poor recovery outcomes in these children as to a desire to escape from their resolute commitments to give care.

Maintenance of hope and positivity

Maintaining a positive outlook despite the perceived tragedy of mental illness and the burden attending an often resolute commitment to give care feature in many of the life stories under study. As in the personal stories, hope and positivity in the face of adversity appears highly valued as a coping response and, once again, may proceed motivationally in terms of maintaining perseverance, here, in carrying out the family caregiving role and in adhering to often troublesome treatment regimes. Also echoing the personal stories, cultural norms may prescribe the voicing of such attitudes toward one's predicament (Pearson and Phillips 1994; Phillips 1993; Xiong *et al*. 1994; Yang and Pearson 2002). Unlike the personal stories, there is little evidence of positive reinterpretation in the family caregiver corpus, the focus of attention for the most part being on the potential gains of the ill family member rather than on those of the caregiver.

Confidence is half of life; it is the fountainhead of one's spiritual support and strength. Not only must you have confidence, but even more important is for you to help your son build confidence …. In sum, I urge you to definitely get rid of any misgivings and build up a steadfast confidence in curing the illness.

[信心是半个生命, 是一个人的精神支柱和力量的源泉. 不仅你要有信心, 更重要的还要帮助你儿子树立信心 … 综上所说, 我劝你一定要消除顾虑, 树立治病的坚强信心.]

(Text XI, Yao 2000, 272–273)

Nowadays my mood remains steady and I live life positively and optimistically, patiently caring for my child. My positive mood has affected my child; he is gradually becoming not so pessimistic. Seeing my now tall and handsome son, my heart is brimming with hope.
[如今, 我的情绪稳定, 积极乐观地生活, 耐心护理孩子. 孩子受我良性情绪的影响, 逐渐的也没有那么悲观了, 看着现在高大英俊的儿子, 我心里充满了希望.]

(Text XIX, Yao 2000, 299)

I have to properly adjust my attitude and firmly believe that, after the storm has past, there, once again, will be a bright tomorrow.
[我要调整好自己的心态, 坚信暴风雨过后, 将又是一个灿烂的明天.]

(Text XXIII, Yao 2007, 93)

Role of society in 'recovery' of the ill family member

As in the personal corpus, many of the family caregivers emphasise 'returning to society' [回归社会; 重返社会] as a primary goal of recovery for the ill family member. They view assisting the ill family member to attain this goal as a key element of their caregiving duties. Recovery from mental illness is highly socially mediated, evidenced through the person with mental illness successfully re-establishing everyday social contact, re-engaging in social activity and contributing to society through productive work or similar activities. Thus, at the core of recovery lies achieving social functioning, with improved quality of life for the person with a mental illness (as determined by the individual) and personal achievements (as defined by the individual), for the most part, being neglected.

Hard work pays off. Through the aforesaid efforts, my son's solitude and laziness took a turn for the better. He now gets along normally with others in his life and at work, and his capacity for social interaction has basically recovered to pre-illness levels.
[功夫不负有心人. 通过上述努力, 我儿的孤独、懒散情况有新好转, 在生活、工作中与人相处正常, 其社会交往能力已基本上恢复到病前水平.]

(Text VII, Yao 2000, 264–265)

We tried hard to create a cosy and peaceful living environment for our child and to actively lead our child into society and the wider world.
[我们努力给孩子创造一个舒适、安静的生活环境, 积极引导孩子走进大自然、走进社会.]

(Text X, Yao 2000, 272)

To date, my son has been working continuously for three and a half years. He has a monthly income. The facts prove that returning to society is very important to the recovery of the ill person. Earning a living can increase confidence in his or her conduct in life.

[到现在, 儿子已连续工作3年半了, 月月有收入. 事实证明回归社会对病人的康复非常重要, 自食其力能增加他们做人的自信.]

(Text XXVII, Yao 2007, 104)

In recovery, society at once constitutes a positive motivational force and a barrier for family caregivers. In the life stories under study the intense stigma against mental illness prevailing in mainland Chinese society remains a pressing concern for many caregivers and their families. It manifests in the prejudiced views toward mental illness held by neighbours, work colleagues or an undifferentiated wider community. People with a mental illness are seen as troublesome 'madmen' [疯子] (Text I, Yao 2000, 241), lacking employment and marriage prospects. They are a 'burden to society' [社会的包袱] and considered to be social 'trash' [废物] (Text III, Yao 2000, 251). They and their families are tainted and pitied, leading to immense loss of face.[7]

The cost is precisely to me and my husband's face. 90 per cent of all the people in our neighbourhood know us. [The news of] 'our son becoming a fool' will rapidly blow like the wind across the entire neighbourhood and onto other acquaintances. After thinking it over a little I decided to trade away my face for my son's health!

[代价就是我和老伴的面子, 整个小区90%的人都认识我们, "儿子傻了"会像风一样迅速吹遍全小区和其他熟人. 稍作思索后, 我决定, 用面子换儿子的健康!]

(Text XXVIII, Yao 2007, 108).

So stigmatised is mental illness in Chinese culture that some family caregivers see it as acceptable and justified. The phenomenon is understandable and reasonable given the disease symptomatology and based on 'historical' grounds.[8] Rarely is stigma vigorously contested by caregivers. Many actively conceal their family member's illness from outsiders (including relatives who are not co-resident and even health professionals) (Yip 2007), in the knowledge that their actions – such as tampering with prescribed medication or refusing in-patient hospital treatment to avoid 'exposing' the ill family member and the family – may be detrimental to the ill family member and so, ultimately, to themselves. Moreover, they view part of the caregiving role as helping the ill family member to accommodate and adapt to social stigma, normalising it in his or her life.

After arriving at the university [my son] experienced discomfort that was impossible to explain: chest pain, anxiety, fear and frequent urination. He was immediately admitted to the university hospital where the doctors diagnosed 'myocarditis' …. Yet the truth could not be divulged. Once the university and his classmates knew that he was mentally ill, it would mean that it all would be over for him. Thus, I was either in for a penny or in for a pound. Apart from the fluids that had to be infused, I stopped giving him all the medicine and tablets prescribed by the hospital and replaced them with the medication used to control his mental illness. But this was taking a huge risk, as I did not know whether the antipsychotic medication and the medication in the infused fluids were contraindicated. If they were, the consequences would be too dreadful to contemplate.

[到校后就感到胸闷、紧张、恐惧、尿频, 说不出的难受. 随即住进了校医院, 医生诊断为"心肌炎" ... 实情还不能相告, 一旦学校和同学们知道他是精神病人, 将意味着他一切都完了. 于是, 我一不做二不休, 除液体不能不输外, 把医院开的药水、药片全部停掉, 换成治精神病的药, 但这要冒很大的风险, 我不知道抗精神病药和所输液体内的药有无矛盾, 一旦有了矛盾, 后果不堪设想.]

(Text I, Yao 2000, 242–243)

Since in our minds we subconsciously thought 'allowing our son to be hospitalised is tantamount to making his condition public, which would see us lose face and would be detrimental to our son's future', we were not willing for our son to be admitted to hospital. And so, after his medication was prescribed, we insisted on treating him back at home.

[由于我们脑海里藏着"让儿子住院等于病情公开, 我们脸面不好瞧, 对儿子今后也不利"的潜意识, 所以不肯让儿子住院, 而坚持开药后回家服药.]

(Text XII, Yao 2000, 277)

Prejudice and discrimination against mentally ill people is caused by the characteristics of this kind of illness and historical reasons. We firstly need to meet this problem head on, that is to say we need to be mentally prepared for it ….

We are trapped by this whole problem of social discrimination; it weighs heavy on our minds. Even though we tried hard to approach it properly, in the process of job placement on graduation we still undertook to conceal my son's medical history as much as possible. We also have not revealed his medical history to his new workplace.

[对精神病人的偏见和歧视是由于这种病的特点和历史原因造成的, 对这个问题我们首先要正视, 也就是说要有思想准备 ... 对于这一社会歧视问题, 我们也存在着困惑, 承受着沉重的思想负担, 在毕业分配过程中, 尽管我们努力正确对待, 但仍是在尽量隐瞒病史的基础上进行的, 在新的工作单位也没有暴露病史.]

(Text XIII, Yao 2000, 279)

Biomedical intervention

As with the personal corpus, the biomedical voice has somewhat low positive resonance in the family caregiver stories, despite their psychoeducational context of publication. Once again, the biomedical voice in the family caregiver corpus is characteristically authoritative in tone, with medication compliance and adherence to directives of the mental health professional highly valued. This occurs despite the fact that family caregivers frequently have to deal with the consequences of pharmacotherapeutic failure, residual symptomatology and untoward medication side-effects.

> People with this kind of illness generally lack insight and most of them are unwilling to take medication according to medical advice. My son is no exception …. We obtained the medication from the hospital and brought it home for him. My husband specifically took care of this and, according to the doctor's advice, divvied up the medication one-by-one, day-by-day, making sure that my son took them on time … Seeing him suffer from the side-effects of taking medication really distressed us. Moreover, urging him to take his medication was difficult work and several times we thought about letting him reduce or stop taking his medication on his own accord. But on thinking deeply about this over and over again we felt that, in order to cure his illness and in the long-term interests of him and his family, no matter how much pain he suffered for the time being and the size of the difficulties faced, we definitely cannot waver in his taking medication according to the doctor's opinion.
> [此类病人一般都缺乏自知力, 大多数都不肯就医服药, 我儿也不例外 … 我们从医院替他取药回来, 由老伴专人保管, 并遵医嘱逐日逐次分好, 按时督促他吃下去 … 我们见他因吃药副作用带来的痛苦实在心疼, 加之劝他吃药工作难做, 曾几次想让他自动减药或停药, 但思考再三, 觉得为了他的病好, 为了他和家庭的长远利益, 不管暂时受到多大痛苦, 遇到多大困难, 遵照医师意见服药决不能动摇.]
>
> (Text VII, Yao 2000, 262)

> Later on we changed to Chlorpromazine. The first time she took it her condition became even more serious. The next morning she appeared extremely agitated with a screaming headache and throwing things around. She took revenge on her mother, forcing me to take her medication, saying it was poison. It made her feel unbearably sick. That very day she began to get a fever, dizziness and nosebleed …. She carried on like this from morning till night, yet I still insisted that she take the medication …. At present she is still in the phase of adjusting the medication and her symptoms are still not yet under control.
> [后来换了氯丙嗪, 吃第一次时, 病情更加严重, 第二天早上出现极度兴奋、大喊头痛、摔东西、报复母亲, 逼母亲吃她的药, 说药是毒药, 使她难受得受不了. 这一天她开始发烧、头晕、鼻出血 … 就这样从早闹到晚, 我还是坚持给她吃了药 … 目前, 她还处于调药阶段, 症状仍未控制.]
>
> (Text XVIII, Yao 2000, 293–294)

Explanatory models of mental illness

In contrast to the personal corpus, the biomedical aetiological explanation for mental illness is often drawn on in the family caregiver stories to explain illness-related behaviours and circumstances. There is only rare engagement of the psychosocial aetiological explanation. There are no instances of multiple explanatory models being simultaneously embraced by family caregivers.

> Looking at it now, if back then we had had the knowledge and experience in this area and had only carefully observed and analysed, then from a few small clues we would have discovered inklings of his schizophrenia. For instance, when he was at home on leave from school, he lost interest in everything, lost confidence also in life, was unwilling to listen to anyone, was overly sensitive and keyed up all day long, with the littlest slip-ups by other people making him angry. This was all directly related to his cognitive reversal. Most typical was his saying that 'in the future I'm either going to die or I'm going to kill someone.'
> [现在看, 如果当时我们具备这方面的知识和经验只要用心观察分析, 就会从一些蛛丝马迹中发现他精神分裂的端倪. 比如他休学在家, 对一切都失去了兴趣, 对生活也失去了信心, 对谁都不愿理睬, 敏感性特强, 整天精神紧张, 别人稍不慎就会触怒他, 这都与他的认知逆转有直接的关系, 最典型的是他说"将来我要么去死, 要么去杀人".]

(Text XII, Yao 2000, 277)

> However, compared to all the losses brought about by a relapse, can persevering in using medication, once again, be regarded as anything much? Don't some other chronic diseases, such as hypertension and diabetes, all require one to continue using medication for the long-term or even lifelong? For this reason we were happy to accept this reality and kept strictly using medication.
> [但是, 与复发带来的各方面的损失相比, 坚持用药又算得了什么呢? 一些别的慢性病如高血压、糖尿病等, 不是都需要坚持长期甚至终生用药吗? 因此我们欣然接受了这个现实, 严格维持用药.]

(Text XIII, Yao 2000, 279)

Comprehensive understanding

Following the analysis undertaken in Chapter 2, the meanings expressed in people's life stories of family caregiving in mental illness are now examined in terms of how they are shaped by culture. This entails consideration of and illustration by means of the temporal and causal ordering of life events, claiming and refashioning of identities, and language use.

Mental illness in the family caregiver stories, once again, constitutes a temporal juncture in the person's life, marking out a life that had met the person's expected life path and one that is now changed for ever. The 'biographical disruption' (Bury 1982, 169) in the family caregiver life stories is even greater than that recounted in the personal stories, commonly drawing on metaphors of not just battle but natural disaster to express the degree of catastrophe and loss experienced. The latter metaphor alludes to the profound effort and resolute commitment required to rebuild and reconstruct what are now commonly seen as broken lives and futures. The significance of the intensity of the language used to describe the tragedy of mental illness is heightened when the psychoeducational context of the stories is taken into account: one may have expected such a context to lead to moderation, by the author or the newsletter editor, of the presentation of the depth of burden and challenge attending family caregiving in mental illness.

Culture shapes this level of catastrophe assigned to mental illness by family caregivers, through the intense stigma against mental illness mentioned in Chapter 2. Familial and social order and harmony are fundamental to Confucian teachings and people with a mental illness are seen as a direct threat to this (King and Bond 1985; Kung 2001; Lin, Tseng and Yeh 1995; Metzger 1981). They are unable to fulfil culturally prescribed roles (Kleinman *et al.* 2011) and their behaviour can be problematic and socially disruptive (Kohrman 2005; Pearson 1996). Of particular concern to families is that a person with a mental illness 'pollutes' a family's genetic line in a culture where patrilineal continuity remains highly valued (Dikötter 1998; Yip 2007). These cultural conceptions are reinforced in contemporary mainland China by a government that views mental illness 'as an organic lesion, a blot on the brain or a hereditary trait that is almost incurable' (Dikötter 1998, 139). The government vigorously and unapologetically promotes eugenic policies directed against many disorders including mental illness, most notably as part of its one-child policy (Dikötter 1998; Pearson 1995b). Cultural and state discourses, thus, coalesce (Holroyd 2001) to emphasise the burden and social challenge mental illness places on family caregivers.

Building on Goffman's seminal definition (see Chapter 2), Link and Phelan (2001, 367) view such stigma as a meeting of 'interrelated' phenomena, namely:

> In the first component, people distinguish and label human differences. In the second, dominant cultural beliefs link labeled persons to undesirable characteristics – to negative stereotypes. In the third, labeled persons are placed in distinct categories so as to accomplish some degree of separation of 'us' from 'them'. In the fourth, labeled persons experience status loss and discrimination that lead to unequal outcomes. Finally, stigmatization is entirely contingent on access to social, economic, and political power …. Thus, we apply the term stigma when elements of labeling, stereotyping, separation, status loss, and discrimination co-occur in a power situation that allows the components of stigma to unfold.

The life stories under study demonstrate this phenomenological convergence, first, with ill family members commonly labelled as 'patients' or 'invalids' [病人] or 'sufferers' [患者], similar to the labels people with a mental illness had applied to themselves in their own life stories. Second, as already noted, cultural stereotypes characterise people with a mental illness as disembodied, disruptive and 'polluted'. This is borne out, and not universally resisted, in the life stories. Third, the illness labels linked with negative cultural stereotyping diminish the personhood of the people with a mental illness, separating them from mainstream society. They need to battle to return to this society. As a consequence, family caregivers take on the responsibility of returning the people they now care for to a society that the people were once members of but now remain excluded from. Fourth, the labels linked with negative cultural stereotyping also locate people with a mental illness in a subordinate position as family members assist them to regain social functioning. The people are detached from personal decision-making and discriminated against in terms of the job market and the marriage pool, unable to enjoy rights (self-determination, employment and reproduction) commonly enjoyed by 'healthy' citizenry. Finally, their disempowered position is legitimised through state policy and legislation that promote the virtues of a eugenic vision and social stability (Bakken 2000; Dikötter 1998).

Link *et al.* (2004, 513) add to this framework the 'emotional responses and reactions' to cultural stigma, broadly equating to Scambler's (2004, 33) notion of '*felt stigma*' encompassing '*shame*' and 'the *fear of encountering enacted stigma*' (for example, overt discrimination by members of the public) (original emphasis).[9] This encourages the concealment of the stigmatised condition from others (Kleinman *et al.* 2011; Lam *et al.* 2011) and the following of protracted pathways to medical care, both documented in the life stories under study. Yang and Pearson (2002, 237) state that such behaviour by Chinese family caregivers only feeds a vicious cycle in that '[t]he more the family is compelled to hide the existence of the [mental] illness, the greater the shame and perceived stigma become.'

The intensity of the stigma attending mental illness in Chinese culture leaves family caregivers in the life stories under study with few 'resources available to them to resist or rework the cultural meanings of [mental] illness' (Kleinman 1988, 26). Many simply accommodate and adapt to the stigma, normalising it in their lives. As such, family caregiving in mental illness becomes an unending struggle against personal loss and the consequences of cultural stigma. The ongoing nature of the caregiving endeavour and the inescapable disruption it brings to caregivers' planned futures contribute to an absence of clear resolution in the stories in question. Returning to society in a productive capacity (recovery) represents a distinct, albeit problematic to achieve, resolution in the life stories of people with a mental illness. The continuing supervision and guidance that characterises family caregiving in the life stories under study, however, must extend beyond any apparent recovery by the person with a mental illness. Where supervision and guidance is neglected following an apparent recovery by the person with a mental illness in the family caregiver stories, relapse invariably ensues. Such a 'lack of an "ending"' in a story of illness, Hydén (1997, 61) observes, leaves storytellers 'forever in search of meaning.' The absence of a clear resolution in the family caregiver stories under study finds most family caregivers seeking out meaning by way of their pasts, revisiting and reaffirming culturally valued identities and roles that they had previously enacted. Notions of nurturing and guardianship (childrearing) are frequently invoked in the stories, providing a sense of continuity between past and present amidst the external challenges faced (Charon 2006). The performance of the family caregiving role, thus, echoes childrearing, as shaped by the dominant cultural script, in that full consideration and commitment are given to protecting ill family members (Yang and Kleinman 2008) and nurturing them toward an envisioned future of productivity in society. At the same time, culture and biomedicine seemingly 'collude' as in the personal stories of mental illness, in designating medication compliance as an essential ingredient in achieving this goal (Ng *et al.* 2008a, 2008b, 2011).

As a consequence, in the stories in question, family caregivers equate success to an ability to ensure that the ill family member is well cared for and protected; that his or her behaviour is agreeable and not socially disruptive; that he or she fully complies with professionally prescribed therapeutic regimes and does not 'relapse'; and that he or she regains full social functioning. They feel obligated to carry out their role with utmost rigour and forbearance, lest the ill family member not achieve a full recovery. Failure to do so serves as a foremost source of guilt and labels them as 'incompetent'. Family caregiving in mental illness thus becomes, as Hydén (1995, 67) states 'a fundamental moral challenge.' The moral challenge lies in meeting the cultural expectations of the family caregiving role. Family caregivers, therefore, commonly blame themselves in the life stories under study for any perceived failures in meeting these expectations, ahead of blaming the illness itself (despite the psychoeducational context of publication of the stories) or the actions of the ill family member. Moreover, the self is blamed rather than questioning the expectations of the caregiving role. Cultural norms prescribe that order must be maintained and that it is the family caregiver's moral responsibility to do so by rigorously monitoring the behaviour of the person being cared for and ensuring medication compliance (Pearson and Lam 2002). This is underscored by state legislation in mainland China which compels families to ensure that people with a mental illness are appropriately cared for and kept under control (Ran *et al.* 2005; Yang and Pearson 2002; Yip 2007). These expectations are never challenged in the life stories under study, and only in extreme, untenable circumstances, such as repeated acts of violence by the ill family member, are cultural (and legal) obligations abandoned. In such cases, the cultural shame arising from the loss of family integrity due to the violence must outweigh the cultural shame arising from abandonment of the obligation to give care.

The weight of cultural expectation causes any notion of empowered subjectivity in the life stories under study to seemingly dissolve as family caregivers carry out their role 'at all costs', including costs to self. A culturally shaped devotion 'to others without thought of self' (Bakken 2000, 105) morally silences resistance to their circumstances or consideration of ways to reduce their burden in family caregiving. Heroic displays of selflessness hold particular salience in mainland China, where the population is well versed in tales of self-sacrifice by modern-day communist heroes such as Lei Feng (Bakken 2000). In the life stories under study, selflessness also appears to deny family caregivers the opportunity to positively reinterpret the challenges they face as gains in personal achievement or self-efficacy. In evidence in the personal corpus, positive reinterpretation remains largely unvoiced in the family caregiver counterpart. Lefley (1996) reports that positive reinterpretation is well documented and positively valued in family caregiving in mental illness in the West. In the life stories under study, disempowerment also stems from family caregiver deference to the health professional, both in terms of following directives, for example, ensuring medication compliance despite less than optimal pharmacotherapeutic outcomes; and in language use, for example, their frequent use of labels such as 'patients' or 'invalids' [病人] and 'sufferers' [患者]. This, too, is shaped by cultural norms of behaviour, which prescribe acquiescence to professional authority and direction (Kleinman 1980; Ramsay 2008), as noted in Chapter 2.

In contrast to the personal corpus, the biomedical aetiological explanation of mental illness is commonly drawn on in the family caregiver counterpart. Despite the potentially problematic intersection of biomedicine and culture-based stigma, proffered as explanation for the minimal voicing of the biomedical aetiological explanation in the personal corpus, the caregivers appear more willing to locate the cause for the family member's disembodiment and problematic behaviours, and the circumstances that follow on from this, in the pathophysiology of illness. Mental illness, for example, is likened to physical illness like diabetes (Barrett 1996; Lafrance 2007; Yamashita and Forsyth 1998). Cultural stigma shapes many aspects of the family caregiver stories, as discussed earlier. However, a confluence of circumstances likely allows the biomedical aetiological explanation to be voiced in the family caregiver stories, despite the potential intersection with cultural stigma. Family caregivers are one step removed from the illness, in not being a sufferer. In the personal stories, people have sought to distance themselves from the culturally shaped idea that, by having mental illness, they have polluted their family bloodline. So they likely shy away from engaging the biomedical aetiological understanding that potentially draws attention to this. Family caregivers, however, do not face this immediate concern of those who are ill. Moreover, the family caregivers are speaking to a newsletter community that likely serves as a support group of fellow family caregivers in mental illness. It would be less problematic to raise the biomedical aetiological explanation with such a group than to raise it with outsiders (mental illness is commonly concealed from relatives and health professionals in the life stories under study). In addition, the family caregivers may perceive a need to acknowledge the biomedical aetiological explanation in their life stories to demonstrate to the newsletter community a full commitment to biomedical reasoning, in line with the life stories that had preceded theirs (Ayometzi 2007; Brody 2003; Garro and Mattingly 2000a). Besides, effecting control over circumstances features in the life stories under study, with biomedical reasoning, namely, pharmacotherapeutic compliance, an essential element in this control.

Conclusion

Analysis of the mainland Chinese life stories of family caregiving in mental illness has documented how culture shapes the temporal and causal ordering of life events, the identities claimed and refashioned, and language use in the stories. Cultural forces, in particular the intense stigma against mental illness in Chinese culture and cultural expectations of normative family caregiving, lead family caregivers to recount mental illness as temporally disruptive and calamitous, with past identities and roles re-engaged in order to carry out family caregiving at all costs. The immoderate language employed to describe mental illness and the uncompromising approach to family caregiving recounted in the life stories, while culturally compliant, would countermand the psychoeducational context of publication of the life stories. Psychoeducation presents a more reasoned and judicious picture of mental illness and emphasises concern for self within the family caregiving endeavour (Xiang *et al.* 1994; Xiong *et al.* 1994; Yip 2005; Zhang *et al.* 1993; Zhang *et al.* 1994).

Nevertheless, as in the personal stories of mental illness analysed in Chapter 2, culture and biomedicine also, at times, shape the family caregiver stories in similar directions. Cultural expectations in recovery entail returning to a productive role in society and biomedicine provides the means by which this is achieved, namely, pharmacotherapy (Ng *et al.* 2008a, 2008b, 2011). Cultural norms prescribe acquiescence to professional authority and direction (Kleinman 1980; Ramsay 2008) and biomedicine valorises medication compliance (Lam *et al.* 2011; Ng *et al.* 2008). Also similar to the personal corpus, the life stories analysed in the current chapter are culturally shaped in ways that provide a sense of comfort to the storyteller. A degree of certainty and continuity is offered in many of the caregivers' disrupted lives by re-engaging past identities grounded in childrearing. A familiar self from before is restored in the present self. Solace is also found in fulfilling the cultural expectation to resolutely give care. The price of this comfort, once again, is disempowerment. A sense of future new selves do not emerge in the stories told (Bury 2001; Frank 1998; Hawkins 1999; Hydén 1997). There is little room for renegotiating the family caregiving role based on individual circumstances. Moreover, family caregiver authority and voice is often ceded in the life stories under study to the health professional and biomedicine.

In sum, this chapter's analysis of life stories of family caregiving in mental illness complements the analysis of the personal stories of mental illness undertaken in Chapter 2. The analysis has identified and considered similarities and differences in how culture shapes the two corpora of life stories. Brody (2003, 129) has called on researchers to 'move away from first-person narratives of the sickness experience in order to hear the stories as told from others' viewpoints.' The next chapter, therefore, examines filmic stories of mental illness recounted in two contemporary mainland Chinese films. In so doing, we can arrive at an understanding of how culture shapes Chinese people's stories of mental illness told from both inside and outside of the experience.

4 Filmic stories of people with a mental illness

This chapter examines how culture shapes stories of people with a mental illness recounted in two contemporary mainland Chinese films, *Baober in Love* [恋爱中的宝贝] and *I Love You* [我爱你]. The value of examining filmic stories, where the account is commonly told from outside of the life experience, is that the prevailing meta-narrative that circulates in a cultural community may be more clearly identified (see Chapter 1). This meta-narrative communicates a culturally dominant view of mental illness, aspects of which may remain hidden from view in life stories told by those inside the experience.

The two films under study, *Baober in Love* and *I Love You*, were released in 2004 and 2002, respectively. The plots of both films are based around the experience of heterosexual love between two young people in contemporary Beijing. In both films, this love is complicated by the existence of mental illness in the female partner. Mental illness, therefore, constitutes a visible subplot in both films, serving to augment and amplify the films' primary plot of life and love in contemporary urban China. The visibility of the mental illness subplot and the contemporaneity of the films in question drove their selection for analysis.

Knight (2006) has observed that the names of mainland Chinese films often incorporate the expression 'love' where social, and so by implication, political critique is being undertaken. This is to 'assert the film's [political] innocence' and so minimise the potential for political repercussions or censorship (Knight 2006, 99). The subplot of mental illness, too, has often been employed 'to symbolise broader social dysfunction' in mainland Chinese literary works of the past which have engaged in political critique (Ramsay 2008, 30). This dates back to the first Chinese modern work of fiction published in 1918, *Diary of a Madman* [狂人日记], written by renowned twentieth century author Lu Xun [鲁迅] (Brassington 1995; Linder 2011; McDougall and Louie 1997; Rojas 2011).

The ensuing analysis focuses not on the social and political critique contained in the films under study but on how the stories of the two female characters with mental illness are culturally shaped (Bhugra 2006). The analysis proceeds by separating out the individual stories of the two women from the broader plots of each of the films and then examining how culture shapes these stories. In like manner to Chapters 2 and 3, this entails consideration of the meanings that emerge through the temporal and causal ordering of life events, through the claiming and refashioning of identities, and through language use. The analysis distinguishes the commonalities in and differences between how culture shapes the life stories of mental illness analysed in the earlier chapters and how culture shapes the filmic stories of mental illness analysed in the current chapter (Hydén 1997). The ensuing analysis also identifies the prevailing meta-narrative of mental illness circulating in Chinese communities, which is drawn on in the films under study (Bordwell 1985; Branigan 1992; Chouinard 2009; Knight 2006; Lothe 2000; O'Shaughnessy and Stadler 2008; Wedding, Boyd and Niemiec 2005).

Analysis of *Baober in Love*

Baober in Love is a 2004 film directed by celebrated 'fifth generation' mainland Chinese female director, Li Shaohong [李少红] (Vanderstaay 2011). The 'fifth generation' is arguably the most well-known group of mainland Chinese film directors, including the likes of male directors Zhang Yimou [张艺谋] and Chen Kaige [陈凯歌]. They are characterised by having lived through the cultural revolutionary period (1966–1976) and having directed films that gained global recognition as mainland China 'opened its doors' to the world post-1978. Their films usually present a critical view of Chinese culture and history, and are commonly regarded as progressive in social outlook, at least to a limit allowed by state censorship.

The film *Baober in Love* explores the effects of rapid industrialisation and modernisation in modern-day Beijing, critiquing 'the negative impact which [this] has on characters who are not mentally equipped to survive the changes' (Vanderstaay 2011, 101). The film centres on the lives of and the emergent relationship between two protagonists: Baober [宝贝], a young woman with a mental illness, and her neighbour and eventual lover, Liu Zhi [刘志], a young professional man disenchanted with his bourgeois lifestyle. The issue of Baober's mental illness, while important in the film, particularly at its tragic conclusion, nevertheless remains subordinate throughout the film to the primary critique of rapid urban industrialisation and modernisation noted above.

Baober's story

The story of Baober in the film *Baober in Love* begins in a primary school classroom. Baober is reciting an essay entitled 'My Birth' [我的出生], these four Chinese characters clearly written in large font on the blackboard. Even though Baober is standing at a focal point in the classroom, located at the front of the central aisle, all her classmates' attention is on the teacher who appears to be giving a lesson. No one, including the teacher, takes any interest in Baober and her tale. The class recesses in the middle of Baober's speech, but she continues on, for the most part undaunted. The image of an isolated figure, thus, emerges from the outset of the film. Moreover, a source of Baober's isolation is already suggested by the narrative prominence that Baober's birth story is given and the camera focus on the Chinese characters for 'birth' written on the blackboard. Baober's 'problem', it seems, is one whose origins can be traced back to her birth.

Baober's story then proceeds back in time to this birth. It takes place, symbolically, in a pile of garbage in the street somewhere in the suburbs of Beijing. In one of the many magic realist sequences that characterise this film, on the night of Baober's birth a meteor trails across the night sky and streaks across the top of her head. Fireworks concurrently erupt. Baober feels as if she were 'a small star dropped onto Earth from the heavens' [我是天上掉落在地球上的一颗小星星]. At this time, Baober's mother is said to have picked newborn baby Baober up from the garbage pile [在垃圾堆拾起我], but not before the newborn is attacked by an alley cat as she lies alone in the garbage pile. The attack by the alley cat, a motif that recurs throughout Baober's life, alongside Baober's atypical and degraded place of birth and the supernatural events that coincided with this birth, together mark Baober as a sullied, strange and extraordinary figure. She has been tainted by a force (mental illness) that will stay with, and likely plague her, throughout her life.

Part of Baober's disturbing persona from an early age is her grating scream, which intrudes throughout the story of her life, in particular whenever she is confronted by her own madness; and which serves to disrupt any sense of sympathy we may have developed for Baober at that point of the story. It is first heard when she is attacked by the alley cat as a newborn. It is next heard when the story returns to her primary school days and the cat motif reappears, a classmate maliciously throwing a cat at Baober one day after class as she leaves the school building. Even at a young age, those in Baober's community actively taunt and bully her, drawing on the nominal symbol of her taintedness: the cat. The scream returns as the young Baober stands in the centre of her home as it is demolished by a demolition crew. She stands there alone, paralysed by fear as the demolition continues. She appears incapable of taking action to stop the demolition and no one offers her aid. She is left isolated, having to face her fear alone without support from her family or others. Immediately after the home is demolished, high-rise apartments that characterise present-day Beijing sprout up from the ground toward the sky, surrounding Baober. She appears dysphoric and unable to make sense of her dislocation.

Baober's story then moves to her teenage life, during the early open-door reform period post-1978, when drabness and uniformity in dress was the norm. For a moment Baober appears one of the crowd, with only subtle, yet noticeable, differences in attire from those around her on the street riding bicycles. This momentary assimilation of Baober into the throngs on the roadway, however, is quickly shattered when she carelessly rides headfirst into a public bus crossing at an intersection, which all the other bicyclists managed to negotiate without much difficulty. We subsequently move to Baober as an adult, where she shifts from an unthreatening figure of derision to one that is unpredictable and socially transgressive and disruptive. While as a younger girl Baober's 'problem' leads to distancing and scorn from those around her, as an adult she becomes a threat. Baober's infatuation with a married neighbour, for example, leads her to force her way uninvited into the neighbour's apartment when his wife is home alone, where she proceeds to impudently scrutinise the various rooms of the lavish apartment. The wife is both taken aback by Baober's effrontery and upset by a video that Baober gives her that purports duplicity and infidelity on behalf of the woman's husband, with whom Baober is infatuated. Baober violates this person's space and, in so doing, cultural norms, in a manner that is strangely detached, carefree and unconcerned.

Baober's emergent transgressive behaviours continue as the story recounts her relationship with an imagined father. She makes initial contact with the elderly demented man when she enters the stranger's home uninvited, asks for a drink and then proceeds to cook a meal there. For the first time we see the formation, albeit manufactured through madness, of a warm social bond between Baober and another person. They seem to connect through their mutual experiences of marginalised worlds, with the demented man reflecting on verse from the 1927 poem by Zhu Ziqing [朱自清], *Moonlight Over the Lotus Pond* [荷塘月色], which celebrates solitude and the embracing of one's individual world. This moment of warmth and connection between the two is short-lived, however, with the demented man collapsing in Baober's company, as she is thinking 'I want to be together with you forever' [我要永远和你在一起].

We next see Baober visiting the old man in hospital, falsely claiming to be his daughter. Despite being informed by the doctor in charge that the man has already died, she cheerfully insists on 'visiting' him, decorating his bed with flowers and pet fish. Seemingly oblivious to the man's death, she reads him verse from *Moonlight Over the Lotus Pond*: 'It's like I have transcended my ordinary self and arrived in another world' [我也像超出了平常的自己, 到了另一个世界]. Those like Baober, it seems, live their lives in worlds quite separate from everyday people.

Baober's trangressive behaviour continues, now with her newfound boyfriend: the neighbour with whom she was infatuated and who has now separated from his wife. She and her newfound lover trespass onto a building site where Baober sets off an emergency alarm. Reminiscent of her being chased and taunted by classmates as she left school as a young girl, Baober and her lover are chased by construction workers on the building site, alerted by the alarm that she has set off. Baober's life, it seems, is characterised by dislocation: from her home, from her school and, now, from a place of sanctuary with her lover. She and her lover eventually find a new home in a deserted warehouse but domestic harmony is short-lived, Baober feeling unable to communicate with her boyfriend [不知道怎么跟他说]. She leaves to live rough in the subway like a vagrant.

However, Baober subsequently develops a relationship with an amputee in a wheelchair, who she finds sitting alone on the sidelines as others in wheelchairs play basketball. His role is to pick up the basketballs after the players have left the venue. Reminiscent of her kinship with the demented old man, Baober feels that she 'particularly understands' the amputee [特别了解你] and returns to his home to stay with him. She appears very comfortable with the amputee and assists him in joining in future basketball games at the court. Her relationship with the amputee is only broken when her previous boyfriend tracks her down to the basketball court and she decides to return home with him.

Baober's story moves to a holiday taken by her boyfriend and herself on the coast. Here her trangressive behaviour continues, with the boyfriend and her making love in public on the beach, a breach of cultural values in a sexually conservative Chinese society. The setting of their love making, despite its potentially romantic atmosphere, is strangely cold and detached, featuring dark coastal rocks, a dim evening sky, a cold, steely ocean, and black cliffs in the distance. It does not present an image of warmth or appealing sexuality to the outsider. The couple, in the end, are arrested by the police for their lewd behaviour in public. Baober suffers an acute psychological breakdown in the police station where she and her boyfriend are taken for questioning, crouching alone – in contrast to her boyfriend who is in a crowded holding cell sitting body-to-body with several other arrestees – in the foetal position in the corner of an interview room, unable to communicate coherently with the bemused police officers. Baober's inconsolable distress causes the police to ponder: 'What's to be done with her?' [她怎么办?].

Baober is next found in her parent's home, crouching alone, in a darkened, austere room, her pose and setting very similar to those found at the police interview room immediately before this. Her parents inform her boyfriend, now released from police detention, that 'Now, she can't recognise anyone' [她现在她谁都不认识]. Her father notes that she has been 'like this from an early age' [从小就这样] and that these acute episodes are brought on by trauma. He laments that the duration of these acute episodes of illness are getting longer over time. Baober's parents express little hope for improvement in her condition and plead with the boyfriend to leave her at home with them and move on with his life. Her father cautions that caring for her is extremely troublesome [太麻烦了]. The boyfriend, however, takes her back to the warehouse where they had lived briefly before.

Baober's mental state merely deteriorates further. She becomes indifferent and unresponsive, even to her boyfriend. He comes to speak of Baober's 'world' [你的世界], echoing the language used by Baober and the old demented man to describe their marginalised lives earlier on. Symptoms unmistakably identifiable as psychiatric now come to the fore. Baober obsessively tries to 'clean' her marked body [我要把自己洗干净] in order to stop an undifferentiated 'them' abusing her [我不要你们骂我]. Baober then becomes under the delusion that she is pregnant, her figure, as she views herself in the mirror, being that of a woman in late-term pregnancy. Yet her true figure, as we see her standing in front of the mirror, is non-pregnant. She is clearly paranoid: she feels her parents are wantonly deceiving her by denying her pregnancy and she believes that the alley cat is biding its time to eventually return for her [它等会, 就会出来了].

More ominously, Baober begins to hallucinate that the alley cat has found her and has come to take her baby away [抢走], just as it had come for her at her birth. The implication is that Baober's baby will then be tainted with her 'problem' from birth, realising a heritable cycle of sufferance. However, Baober 'wants a clean child' [我想要一个干净的孩子], free from the stigma she bears. She tries to hide from the cat by covering all the windows in their home with long, dark, thick drapes. Indeed, this guise allows her to capture the cat, seemingly soothing her fears for her baby. This brief relief is dramatically upset, however, in the conclusion of Baober's story when she mortally disembowels herself in what constitutes either a desperate attempt to save herself and her child from their predestined fate, that is, a lifetime of mental illness; or a self-sacrificing act to free her now 'safe' – with the capture of the alley cat – expected child from his or her tainted mother and so release him or her to the world of 'normality'.

Discussion

In contrast to the life stories analysed in the earlier chapters, mental illness does not mark a temporal juncture in Baober's life in the film, but constitutes a taint from birth which manifests throughout the temporal stages of her life: from infancy, through childhood and adulthood, and through to death. Baober is marked at birth, a troubled victim in infancy and childhood, actively transgressive and marginalised in adulthood, and passive but dangerous: approaching her death at her own hands.

What usually constitutes a pure and innocent stage of a person's life, the birth of the baby is recounted as a time of essential contamination of the person with a mental illness. In the film, Baober's birth is portended by mysterious stellar phenomena, an unfavourable omen as to what is to follow. The birth also takes place in a decidedly 'unclean' location, a garbage pile, symbolising (as recounted in Chapter 3) the prevailing cultural view of people with a mental illness as human 'trash'. Any sense of innocence that attends the image of the newborn Baober is taken away in an instant as the newborn is attacked by an alley cat, a recurring symbol of Baober's affliction returning throughout her life in the story.

In childhood, mental illness manifests through Baober's strange aloofness and isolation as she recites the essay in class. This marks her as different, as a troubled 'other'. She is victimised for this, snubbed by her peers and her teacher or actively bullied. At times she appears oblivious to these actions; at other times these actions exclude and distress her. She does not retaliate against these actions. The child with mental illness is seemingly powerless, a receiver of, rather than the purveyor of, harm. This isolation and disempowerment is emphasised by the circumstances of the demolition of her home and the failure of others in society, even her own parents, to rescue her from her trauma. Helplessness and hopelessness, thus, come to characterise the experience of mental illness. Such values are not ascribed to mental illness in the life stories analysed in the earlier chapters.

The teenage years present a fleeting moment of apparent cultural acceptance and assimilation for Baober. Possibly, her unusual behaviours do not mark her as any more out of the ordinary than everyday teenagers. This literally comes to a crashing halt (into a public bus presumably full of 'normal' passengers), with adulthood. Henceforth, Baober's passivity in the face of her culturally shaped marginalisation from society changes to active engagement in acts of social transgression. People with a mental illness in Chinese culture are particularly maligned due to their designation as being disruptive and troublesome (see Chapters 2 and 3). This informs the cultural stigma experienced by Chinese people with a mental illness (Pearson 1996). The adult character of Baober conveys such an image of people with mental illness. Granted, the film's criticism of mainstream modern-day life in Beijing required a transgressive character, but the concomitant identification of the character with mental illness blurs the boundary between social critique and portrayal of the experience of mental illness. In adulthood, Baober's transgressions are frequent and many. She wantonly trespasses, dupes, seduces, forsakes and engages in lewd behaviour. Such behaviours are seldom spoken of in the life stories analysed in the earlier chapters. In the filmic counterpart, however, the adult person with a mental illness unmistakably becomes a purveyor of harm on society and her significant others.

A cost of this for Baober is the deepening cultural isolation and marginalisation that afflicts her in adulthood. As a child, although set apart from her community, Baober still took part in daily social activities, such as attending school and going on beach outings. However, in adulthood she is rarely engaged with the broader community. Adulthood is like colliding with a public bus. The community is disapproving of Baober. She is ignored by clerks in the shopping mall, construction workers chase her from their building site, fellow subway passengers glare at her disapprovingly, and the police view her as problematic. Mental illness is presented as worsening over time.

Baober does find a sense of connection with other marginalised people in society: the demented old man, the amputee and the wheelchair basketball players. People with a mental illness in the life stories analysed in Chapter 2, in like manner, found connection in the community of fellow sufferers. In the end, however, Baober is unable to sustain even these relationships. She also attempts to connect with the mainstream by acting out the normative roles for a woman in Chinese culture, as filial daughter (for a demented stranger), dutiful wife (for an already married man), committed homemaker (in an abandoned warehouse) and devoted mother (for a non-existent expected child) (Cook and Dong 2011; Guo 2010; Roberts 2010). Yet, in the end, these roles turn out to be mere fragile pretences that she cannot sustain. She remains culturally disembodied (Kleinman *et al.* 2011; Traphagan 2000). The person with mental illness, once again, is characterised as helpless and hopeless, progressively deteriorating and ever incapable of functioning in Chinese society.

The end stage of Baober's life is characterised by passivity and danger. She is no longer an active transgressor but, once again, a passive victim. As was the case during the periods of victimhood she experienced as a newborn and a child, Baober is alone and isolated. However, unlike her behaviour during those periods of victimhood experienced as a child, she withdraws totally from society to the confines of her warehouse home and the terror of her psychosis. The culturally resonant theme of hopelessness in mental illness is augmented by the themes of fear and danger (Brassington 1995; Kleinman *et al.* 2011; Linder 2011; Yang 2011).

In this end stage of Baober's life, the Chinese cultural stereotype of a person with mental illness is tragically fulfilled. Baober is acutely psychotic with nobody able to save her from her tragic plight. Not her parents, who play a minimal role in her life but fulfil their cultural obligation to give care when she is acutely ill (see Chapter 3), albeit 'care' that equates to control (locking her up alone in her bedroom) and bears an eerie resemblance to the 'care' proffered to Baober at the police station when she was detained for lewd behaviour. Nor can Baober's boyfriend save her; she has long disengaged from him emotionally and mentally. Ultimately, Baober becomes a danger not to others but to herself. She fatally harms herself (and, in her mind, possibly her expected child as well). The birth-death cycle resonating in this end stage of Baober's life returns us to the beginning of her story.

The beginning and the end of the film under study both call attention to the hereditary nature of mental illness and the view in Chinese culture that it pollutes family lines (see Chapters 2 and 3). The film opens with Baober as a child in primary school reciting an essay at the front of the class. The Chinese characters that title her essay direct us back to her birth [我的出生]. As noted earlier, the film then flashes back to this birth and the contamination of Baober, which is heralded astrologically, signified by location (Baober is lying in a garbage pile), and effected by the alley cat. The alley cat returns at the conclusion of the film, seemingly to secure a similar fate for Baober's expected child, as had befallen herself at birth. Baober's pregnancy, albeit phantom, and the return of the alley cat together serve as reminder of the hereditary nature of mental illness and its stigmatisation in Chinese culture. Baober's exceedingly desperate and ultimately fatal act may be viewed as a natural consequence of her failure to sustain the culturally prescribed roles of daughter, wife, homemaker and mother. Equally, her terminal act may constitute the only means by which the Chinese mother with a mental illness can liberate her child from a genetically-determined cycle of sufferance and life on the margins of society.

In sum, the story casts mental illness as an affliction from birth. The temporal and causal arrangement of life events in the story consistently point back to birth as the origin of the taint of mental illness. The language of Baober's enigmatic essay ('My Birth') and the language of her parents ('[she's been] like this from an early age') reinforce this. Such an aetiological conception of mental illness reflects the prevailing cultural understanding of mental illness and its origins (see Chapters 2 and 3). Mental illness is also cast as threatening, temporally regressive and without hope. Hopelessness is seldom voiced in the life stories analysed in earlier chapters. These stories spoke of recovery and a return to society. In the film, however, the tragic fate of the person with a mental illness is presented as predestined from birth. She will always be 'troublesome', adopting the language of her parents, and be social 'trash', a prominent metaphor made use of in *Baober in Love* and also alluded to in the life stories analysed in Chapter 3. Attempts at 'cleansing' the innate taint of mental illness, either by acting out the normative feminine roles prescribed by Chinese culture or by obsessive bathing of her body, are unable to cleanse the person with a mental illness of this taint and her ultimately fatal lot.

Analysis of *I Love You*

I Love You is a 2002 film directed by well-known 'sixth generation' mainland Chinese male director, Zhang Yuan [张元] (Knight 2006). The 'sixth generation' of mainland Chinese film directors are characterised as 'post-cultural-revolutionary', having grown up during the open-door reform period (post-1978), but having been influenced by the 1989 'June Fourth' Tiananmen incident and its political aftermath throughout the 1990s. Their work is often post-modern in style, engaging in social critique that often deals with urban life in post-Mao mainland China. They pay particular attention to the more individualistic concerns of social alienation and personal satisfaction. Sixth generation film directors are commonly regarded as progressive in their social outlook, but, unlike their fifth generation predecessors, often pay little heed to the limits prescribed by state censorship guidelines and, as a consequence, frequently fall foul of them (Knight 2006).

Zhang Yuan's films, specifically, often consider the lives of stigmatised subaltern groups in mainland China, such as the intellectually disabled, underground musicians, homosexuals and alcoholics (Knight 2006). While the protagonists of *I Love You* are not outwardly marked as subaltern, throughout the film the mental illness of the female protagonist becomes evident. More broadly, the film documents the disintegration of a marriage between two young people lacking in life experience and relationship experience: Du Xiaoju [杜小桔], a young nurse who lost her first fiancé in tragic circumstances, and her husband, Wang Yi [王毅], a young and carefree, but emotionally immature, office worker.

Du Xiaoju's story

Du Xiaoju's story in *I Love You* recounts a much shorter period of time in Du Xiaoju's life when compared to the story of Baober in *Baober in Love*. It largely covers the lead up to Du Xiaoju's marriage, her rocky marriage, the eventual divorce, and the early period post-divorce. Du Xiaoju's past is recounted on occasion throughout the story, but to a much lesser extent and with much less detail than is the case in Baober's story.

The story of Du Xiaoju sets up a sense of intrigue, or 'difference', about Du Xiaoju from the outset. Not at birth, as was the case with Baober, but at a young age nonetheless. During a conversation between Du Xiaoju and her first prospective husband, which leads to a commitment of marriage from him after a very short courtship, she states that she dislikes people calling her by her full name [特讨厌人家叫我全名]. She explains that the reason for this is because her father made her change her family name at a young age, from her father's family name 'Wang' [王] to her mother's family name 'Du' [杜] [我小时候叫王, 因为我爸姓王. 后来我叫杜, 因为我妈姓杜 … 我爸让我改的]. Du Xiaoju then, like Baober, is marked as different from a young age. That this mark of difference taints her is suggested by the subsequent death of the prospective husband in a freak accident. He is killed diving at night into an empty swimming pool that, unbeknownst to him, had earlier been drained for cleaning.

Following her prospective husband's death Du Xiaoju is reunited one day with the deceased man's best friend, at the hospital where she works as a nurse. She spends more time with the man, even though he is dating her girlfriend. On one occasion she allows him to sleep over in her apartment and they make love. Du Xiaoju, therefore, is cast as a morally transgressive and, as such, 'suspect' character. The sense of strangeness about Du Xiaoju, even the inklings of a sense of threat presented by her character, are fortified when she proceeds to use verbatim the same sequence of lines to secure a marriage commitment from her new partner as she had used at the outset of the film to secure one from her now deceased partner. The lines proceed from 'So, am I the one you've always wanted since childhood?' [那我是你从小到大都想要的那个人吗?]. The marriage commitment is obtained, once again, after a very short courtship.

The couple are married and on their wedding night, immediately after Du Xiaoju's girlfriends have left, Du Xiaoju proceeds to repeatedly question her husband about his opinions of one of her girlfriend's appearance. She then repeatedly questions him about his previous female acquaintances' appearances as well as his sexual history: 'Was there anyone better than me, prettier than me?' [有没有比我好的, 长的比我好看的?]. Despite her husband's reassurances she is never consoled.

These behaviours by Du Xiaoju are somewhat disconcerting, but her husband's subsequent behaviour in the early period of their marriage is also immature and provocative. For example, he describes her as 'looking like a whore' [画的跟个鸡似的] after she is made up for free at a cosmetics kiosk in a shopping mall, which leads them to noisily quarrel in public and Du Xiaoju to run off distressed. Nevertheless, that night Du Xiaoju appears strangely unconcerned about the public quarrel with her husband, subsequent to which he had almost been arrested by the police for hooliganism. She is equally nonchalant about her disappearance and subsequent failure to turn up for a dinner planned with her in-laws that evening: 'I didn't want to disgust them, so I went shopping …. [Look,] I bought a new jacket for you.' [我一想算了, 别给人家添堵了自己逛街去了 … 后来啊, 我买了好几件衣服给你买了一件]. Such behaviour would be considered extremely inappropriate in Chinese culture.

Similar events follow, with the marriage becoming increasingly dysfunctional, characterised by constant confrontation, quarrelling, abuse and violence. However, amidst the trauma Du Xiaoju's husband inflicts, her reactions remain perplexing and disturbing. She reacts in an immature manner, is calculating in her provocation, and frequently behaves in a way that is disproportionate to the circumstances. In one instance, she runs away from their apartment just to see how long her husband will search for her: 'I didn't go far at all. I just wanted to see if you'd come looking for me.' [我根本就没走远. 我就想看你想不想找我]. In another example, she is verbally abusive to her husband in public: 'You'd be happy if I never came back home …. Fuck off home!' [你巴不得我永远不回来, 你才高兴呢 … 回屁家!]. Once again, such behaviour would be considered extremely inappropriate in Chinese culture.

As the relationship approaches its lowest point, we hear the first allusion to Du Xiaoju's mental illness, where she ascribes it to her love for her husband [我是脑子进水, 我爱你爱的我脑子进水了]. Following this, instance after instance of Du Xiaoju's transgressive behaviour is recounted. They begin as mild transgressions. Du Xiaoju is wholly unsupportive, in fact mocking, of her husband's failure to be promoted at his workplace: 'What important things can an insignificant employee like you do at work?' [你一个小职员在单位不就这点儿破事吗?]. She brazenly teases her husband about made-up affairs that she has had with more kind, more handsome and richer suitors than he:

> I'll tell you, there are a lot of men chasing me. You may treat me poorly but there are men who treat me well. So many, both inside and outside the hospital. Some more handsome than you, some richer than you. Oh, how come I'm so unlucky to find you? [我告诉你啊, 追我的人可多了. 你对我不好, 可有人对我好. 我这院里院外太多了. 有长的比你好看的, 有比你有钱的. 哎, 我怎么就这么倒楣找到你了].

Du Xiaoju locks her husband out of their apartment and then suddenly unlocks the door as he kicks it in in frustration, so that he falls over. She reacts as if this is just a funny joke. More seriously, Du Xiaoju refuses her husband's request for a divorce then sets fire to their apartment as he tries to leave. She threatens to kill herself and physically barricades the door so he cannot leave. Throughout this Du Xiaoju remains blithely unaware of the gravity of her actions. She believes her behaviour is acceptable since she always apologises afterward: 'At times I like to fight with you? Isn't that because I …. Well, anyway, so don't I usually apologise to you? I have never said that I'm in the right' [我就有时候我爱和你吵架吗? 那还不是因为我 — 对, 再说, 那我不是不是经常跟你认错吗? 我也没说我对啊!]. In the end, Du Xiaoju compromises with her husband's request for a divorce by asking for three more years with her husband, after which she will agree to a divorce [再给我三年吧. 三年之后, 我就让你走].

Du Xiaoju's demeanour deteriorates further from this point on. At this point, she confesses that she is 'mentally unwell' [我是心理上不健康]. In her depths of despair, one day Du Xiaoju ties up her husband on the sofa (where he is now sleeping at night) and holds a butcher's knife to his neck, imploring him to tell her that he loves her. By chance she is called away to tend one of her patients in the hospital ward and he takes the opportunity to sound the alarm by smashing his bound body against a window pane. Du Xiaoju later tells her husband that she regrets not having killed or disfigured him when she had the opportunity to do so [我真想那天一刀下去没把你杀死, 就给你弄一个残废].

Following this act of violence, the couple divorce. At this time, Du Xiaoju is called to visit her ailing father. Her ex-husband accompanies her and discovers that Du Xiaoju's father is, in fact, in prison for having murdered (strangled) her mother 15 years ago. He now lies seriously ill in the prison infirmary, near death. The circumstances underlying Du Xiaoju's change of family name, which so disconcerted Du Xiaoju at the outset of the film, are now explained as an attempt by her father to distance her from his misdeed and the psychopathology that likely contributed to it. The mere changing of a name, however, has not prevented his daughter from repeating the sins of her father, saved only by a chance of fate. It seems Du Xiaoju's state of mind and, so, her destiny, were genetically predetermined.

Du Xiaoju appears very reasonable on her last meeting with her ex-husband following their divorce, but this is short-lived. Afterward, she bicycles wildly the wrong way up a freeway off-ramp, endangering her life. Her ex-husband happens to be driving down the same road and rescues her. She awakes the next day, back in their apartment, to find him by her bedside. She thinks they are still married and cannot understand why he has facial scars from her attack on him. She laments: 'How is it the moment I'm not watching you, you get into trouble?' [我怎么一会儿不看着你, 你就惹事啊?].

The story of Du Xiaoju concludes with the revelation that she is pregnant. The final scene of the film shows Du Xiaoju, divorced and living alone, sitting in a park smiling to herself as she embraces her pregnant abdomen. It is not a warm smile. While Du Xiaoju appears to have found some sense of security in having a child, one is left to contemplate a repetition of Du Xiaoju's (and her father's) suffering, in the life of her newborn.

Discussion

While Du Xiaoju's story in *I Love You* covers a shorter time frame than Baober's in *Baober in Love*, centring on Du Xiaoju's adult married life, there are similarities in the temporal dimensions of the two women's stories of mental illness. In both stories mental illness deteriorates over time, both women in adulthood becoming increasingly culturally transgressive. Events that may exonerate their culpability, in the end, are countermanded by the mounting gravity of the transgressions acted out by the person with a mental illness. Du Xiaoju, more so than Baober, might have been excused for her provocative and calculating behaviours by her husband's insensitivity and self-centredness. Yet Du Xiaoju's final life-endangering actions at a time when her husband's behaviour had become more level-headed largely quell any inclinations to exonerate her, labelling her, like Baober, as a threat.

A genetic aetiology of mental illness is also emphasised in Du Xiaoju's story. Du Xiaoju, like Baober, is marked from birth, in this case by her family name. The misfortune brought on her and those close to her is predestined. Changing a family name will not erase the stain that attends her family history of psychopathology. It is inevitable that she repeats the sin of her father in trying to harm her spouse. The heritable cycle of sufferance is alluded to again at the end of her story, where she is pregnant, divorced and facing an uncertain future. Will her genetic stain be carried on in her expected child?

Du Xiaoju, like Baober, also attempts to connect with the mainstream by acting out the normative roles for a woman in Chinese culture. She is successful for a period of time, contributing to society in her professional capacity as a nurse, viewed as a 'respectable' profession in contemporary mainland China (Guo 2010, 59). She expresses with pride that her 'boss totally trusts me' [领导对 我可放心了]. Du Xiaoju, therefore, temporarily manages to avoid the social isolation and marginalisation that plagued Baober throughout her life. The change of family name and the shame of her father being hidden securely away in a prison hospital would have helped in this. Yet, as culturally expected, the person with a mental illness is incapable of maintaining a functional role in society. Du Xiaoju's obsessive and destructive behaviour as a devoted wife leads her to expose her 'true' state of mind and repeat the sin of her father, saved only by a chance of fate.

Thus, both *I Love You* and *Baober in Love* draw on the prevailing meta-narrative of mental illness circulating in Chinese communities which devalues and stigmatises people with a mental illness. This meta-narrative maintains that mental illness is hereditary and pollutes family lines (Dikötter 1998). It declares that mental illness is regressive and menacing and invariably ends in tragedy (Brassington 1995). It presents people with a mental illness as erratic, morally suspect, social failures and a danger to society (Brassington 1995; Kleinman *et al.* 2011; Linder 2011; Yang 2011; Yang and Kleinman 2008). They are isolated, residing in a different world to mainstream society (Brassington 1995; Lan 2011; Linder 2011; Rojas 2011; Yang 2011).

Most of the characterisations of people with a mental illness which are promulgated by the meta-narrative drawn on in the films analysed in the current chapter, however, remain unvoiced in the life stories analysed in the earlier chapters. They are supplanted in the life stories by more optimistic expectations of the life trajectory and a more integrated, albeit still devalued, social standing for the Chinese person with a mental illness.

In contrast to Knight's (2006) study of the stories of an alcoholic father in the 1996 mainland Chinese film *Sons* [儿子] and a person with cerebral palsy in the 1998 mainland Chinese film *The Common People* [关于爱的故事], no sympathetic counter-narrative of mental illness is proffered in the films analysed in the current chapter. There may be momentary compassion for Baober when she is trapped as a child in her home while it is being demolished and for Du Xiaoju when she is treated poorly by her insensitive husband as a newlywed. This compassion, however, promptly succumbs to bewilderment, antipathy and fear as the two women's mental health progressively deteriorates, culminating in their acts of violence.

One wonders if the meta-narrative of mental illness would have been employed if the protagonists were men, given the more sympathetic account of the alcoholic father in *Sons*, which also was directed by Zhang Yuan (Knight 2006). At times, the father displayed signs of mental illness as well. Being a woman in Chinese culture and having mental illness leave a person doubly subjugated due to the traditionally subordinate roles of Chinese women – which both Baober and Du Xiaoju try to act out in vain – and the intense stigma toward mental illness. Thus, discursively, the meta-narrative of mental illness is more coherent with the gender script for women, as opposed to men, in Chinese culture. What is more, a meta-narrative that promulgates notions of contamination at birth and stained heredity resonates more powerfully through women protagonists. Women, obviously, are the bearers of children and, as such, are physically present as the child is 'marked' from birth.

A discursive link between normative womanhood and mental illness has also been explored in Western cinema. Chouinard (2009) finds in her analysis of 'cultural narratives about the lives and places of women with mental illness in the commercial Hollywood film: *Girl, Interrupted* (1999)' (791) that 'gendered processes of meaning-making' (791) portray 'a more "appropriate" gendered figure of feminine, desirable ways of contending with being a mentally ill woman' (801). A woman with mental illness who can sustain culturally feminine qualities, therefore, has the prospect of being viewed as 'comfortingly ordinary' (Chouinard 2009, 800). Failure to do so leaves her saddled, however, with the prevailing stereotype of being 'disturbingly horrific and other' (Chouinard 2009, 800). The women protagonists in the films analysed in the current chapter, too, seek out a sense of normalcy and self-understanding through the acting out of normative feminine roles in Chinese culture, yet both, in the end, fail in their attempts, leaving them marginalised and 'othered'. Such failure is prescribed by the prevailing meta-narrative of mental illness circulating in Chinese communities. Such failure may also proceed from the women not seeking out professional help and care. In *Girl, Interrupted*, a willingness 'to embrace places of psychiatric care as therapeutic and healing' is a necessary condition for sustaining feminine subjectivity (Chouinard 2009, 802). Such failure may also stem from, as Brassington (1995) finds in mainland Chinese literary works, romantic love for people with a mental illness being culturally taboo. All in all, a 'desirable' and 'comfortingly ordinary' portrayal of a Chinese woman with a mental illness, therefore, becomes unviable in the films in question.

The meta-narrative of mental illness, of course, is drawn on in the films analysed in the current chapter to critique contemporary mainland Chinese urban life and society allegorically. Mental illness merely constitutes a subplot in the films. The directors' purposeful use of this meta-narrative in their films, nevertheless, demonstrates the strength of its cultural resonance, especially when the protagonists are women. The social outlooks, deemed progressive, and genders of the directors of the two films, Li Shaohong, a woman, and Zhang Yuan, a man, add weight to this claim. A meta-narrative that devalues and stigmatises women with a mental illness is wholly uncontested in the contemporary productions at all levels of its expression. This occurs even with a woman director.

Conclusion

Analysis of the filmic stories of the experiences of people with a mental illness has documented how culture shapes the temporal and causal ordering of life events, the identities claimed and refashioned, and the language used in the stories. Mental illness is portrayed as present from birth and deteriorating over time. It results in normative gender roles being sought out but not sustained. The only identity that is sustainable for the person with a mental illness is one of stigmatised 'other' (Harper 2004). Family caregivers remain peripheral to the stories in question but, where depicted, seek to effect control, as recounted in the life stories analysed in Chapter 3.

Both of the films under study draw on the prevailing meta-narrative of mental illness circulating in Chinese communities which devalues and stigmatises people with a mental illness. In this meta-narrative, people with a mental illness are seen as erratic, transgressive and threatening. The meta-narrative maintains that mental illness is hereditary and pollutes family lines. There is no hope for people with a mental illness. The nature of this meta-narrative and of gender scripts in Chinese culture, it is argued, results in little chance of a 'sympathetic' or 'commonplace' account of a Chinese woman with a mental illness being portrayed. Such a portrayal may be viable in Chinese filmic stories of men with a mental illness (Knight 2006) and in Western filmic stories of women with a mental illness (Chouinard 2009).

The negative portrayal of people with a mental illness in the films occurs regardless of the gender of the film director or her or his 'generational' label. This highlights the strength of cultural resonance of the meta-narrative, drawn on in their films to critique contemporary urban life and society in mainland China. Negative and backward-looking portrayals of people with a mental illness, needless to say, also characterise Western films (Birch 2012; Chouinard 2009; Fuery 2003; Wedding *et al.* 2005). The analysis undertaken in the current chapter, nevertheless, identifies the ways in which such a portrayal in the Chinese films is culturally shaped (Bhugra 2006).

In sum, this chapter's analysis of films about people with a mental illness complements the analysis of life stories of mental illness undertaken in Chapters 2 and 3. Analysis of the filmic stories has identified culturally shaped elements unvoiced in the life stories. Thus, an understanding of how culture shapes Chinese people's stories of mental illness told from both inside and outside of the experience has now been provided by this book. In the following chapters we explore further how culture shapes Chinese people's stories of dementia.

5 Life stories of family caregiving in dementia

In Chapters 2 and 3 we explored how culture shapes life stories recounting the experiences of Chinese people with a mental illness and their family caregivers. The current chapter focuses on the experiences of Chinese people caring for a family member with dementia. As a degenerative disorder that afflicts the mind yet, unlike mental illnesses such as schizophrenia and clinical depression, is irreversible, the caregiving experience in dementia takes on particular importance as the family member progressively loses the ability to carry out fundamental human activities such as personal care, eating and drinking, and verbal communication. As a consequence, the life experience of the person with dementia becomes strongly bound to the life experience of their family caregiver. Loss of communicative abilities, in particular, means that any account of the experiences of the person with dementia is usually voiced by others. In Chinese societies, this is commonly the voice of the family caregiver, given that the vast majority of Chinese people with dementia are cared for by family members in the home setting (Au et al. 2010; Gallagher-Thompson et al. 2010; Kleinman 2010; Petrus and Wing-chung 2005).

In the introductory chapter of this book, we saw how economic progress in mainland China and Hong Kong has produced a significantly increased life expectancy and, as a result, a large rise in dementia cases (Au et al. 2010; Ikels 1998; Qiu 2007). Au et al. (2010, 256), for example, estimate that in Hong Kong 'around 60,000 people are living with AD (Alzheimer's disease) today with an estimated prevalence number of 332,000 by 2050'. While family caregiving remains the norm, the Hong Kong regional government now acknowledges the place of institutions in meeting future demand for aged and dementia care (Holroyd 2001). Accordingly, the number of such institutions in Hong Kong is expanding, although questions have been raised about their ease of access and quality (Cheng 2009).[1] The picture in mainland China largely mirrors that of Hong Kong. People with dementia already number around six to seven million (Feng et al. 2011; Qiu 2007; Song and Wang 2010) or 'a quarter of all such patients in the world', with predictions of 'more than 1 million new cases in China every year' (Qiu 2007, 582). The mainland Chinese government now officially acknowledges that dementia, which was previously dismissed 'as a disease of developed countries and so … not an issue in China', now constitutes a pressing concern for contemporary and future society (Qiu 2007, 582). In particular, the one-child policy and internal migration away from rural areas to the urban centres of employment are impacting on the ability of mainland Chinese families to care for the elderly in the home setting. Aged and dementia care facilities do exist in mainland China but, as in Hong Kong, questions have been raised about their accessibility and quality (Gui 2001; Holroyd 2003; Li and Lemke 2004; Zhan 2006).

The family caregiver stories under study in the current chapter were located in two sources. The first source constitutes a collection of family caregiver stories *Don't Leave; Don't Give Up: Voices of Family Members Caregiving for Alzheimer's Disease*[2] *Sufferers* [不離不棄: 老年痴呆症患者家屬照顧心聲], edited by the Hong Kong Alzheimer's Disease Association Publishing Group[3] [香港老年痴呆症協會出版組] and published in 2002 by the Hong Kong Alzheimer's Disease Association [香港老年痴呆症協會] in conjunction with the Hong Kong Society for Rehabilitation Community Rehabilitation Network [香港復康會社區復康網絡]. The edited volume records nine life stories of family caregiving in dementia. The stories recount six women's (two wives and four daughters) and three men's (two husbands and one son) experience of family caregiving in dementia. They range from approximately 2000 to 5000 characters in length (approximating 1500 to 3750 English words). The stories were elicited through interview and later transcribed and reflected on by 'freelance writers' [自由撰稿人] commissioned by the HKADAPG (HKADAPG 2002, i). On average, transcription of the first-person family caregiver account comprises approximately half of an individual life story with third-person freelance writer reflection on what had been recounted at the interview comprising the other half. Thus, on average, around half of a life story is recounted by way of the words of the family caregiver with the other half recounted by way of the words of the freelance writer. There is consistency and coherence between these two perspectives. This is probably unsurprising given that the role of the freelance writer was to elicit and document, rather than critique based on a research or institutional agendum (Cortazzi 1993; Freeman 2004; Hydén 1995; O'Brien and Clark 2010. See Chapter 2), the life stories of Chinese people caring for a family member with dementia in Hong Kong.

The second source of family caregiver stories is the autobiography *Memories Lost and Found*[4] [似曾相識], authored by Lee Hong Ken [李洪根] and published in 2005 by The Universal Press Limited[5] [環球(國際)出版有限公司]. Lee's book recounts his experience of caregiving for his wife with dementia. It is approximately 30,000 characters in length (approximating 22,500 English words). Lee's book, like the HKADAPG volume described above, offers 'testimony' about an experience of illness, in this case, family caregiving in dementia in Hong Kong (Brody 2003; Hawkins 1999). Brody (2003, 113) states that, through such testimony, the person:

> feels healed to the extent that he has attached meaning to his experience
> with his words and his story and to the extent that the act of telling has

reconnected him to his fellow human beings. The community is healed to the extent that they see a fellow person coping with illness and suffering and think that when their time comes, they, too, can find ways to cope and perhaps even to flourish despite illness.

The similar genre of stories published in Lee's book and the HKADAPG volume, together with cultural shaping, provide explanation for the similar linguistic and semantic structures explicated in these stories in the subsequent analysis undertaken in this chapter (see Table 5.1 in the next section of this chapter). This similarity in the language and themes and subthemes characterising the life stories, therefore, occurs regardless of the length of the story and whether the story was recounted solely by the family caregiver, as in the case of Lee's book, or partly by the family caregiver and partly by a third party, as in the case of the HKADAPG volume. This similarity also occurs regardless of whether the story, as in the case of Lee's book, was freely written under the own initiative of and in the own time of the family caregiver, with ample time for reflection on and consideration of the experience of caregiving in dementia; or whether the story was elicited through interview and transcribed by a third party, as in the case of the HKADAPG volume.

As a consequence of the similarity in the linguistic and semantic structural features, the nine life stories from the HKADAPG volume and Lee's life story are combined and analysed together as a single corpus composed of ten stories of family caregiving in dementia. The stories comprising this corpus recount the experiences of Chinese family caregivers residing in urban locations in Hong Kong and whose vocations and home lives point to working and middle class backgrounds. As noted in Chapter 1, the Chinese community in Hong Kong espouse and uphold the same fundamental cultural understandings, norms, values and scripts as their compatriots on the mainland (Chow 2001; Chung 2001; Holroyd 2003; Lam 2006; Petrus and Wing-chung 2005). Nevertheless, in view of Hong Kong's 'unique socio-political history' in being a British colony for one and a half centuries until joining the People's Republic of China in 1997 (Gray *et al.* 2009, 926), the regional context will not be overlooked in the ensuing analysis.

Analysis of family caregiver life stories of dementia

This chapter follows the analytic procedure set out in Chapter 2 in explicating how culture shapes the Hong Kong Chinese life stories of family caregiving in dementia. Similarities to and differences from the mental illness counterparts analysed in Chapter 3 will feature in the ensuing analysis.

Naïve understanding

Family caregivers speak of the sadness attending their loved one's decline, from someone once considered to be a healthy, functional individual to someone whose progressively increasing and worsening deficits result in her or him returning to what resembles a childlike state. This decline serves as an inescapable reminder to the caregiver of the impending demise of the ill family member. Family caregivers, therefore, mourn the loss of the person who they knew in health while, to a certain extent, also grieving ante-mortem in anticipation of the death of the 'altered' person who they now care for. This person is expected, by necessity, to passively accede to the demands of the family caregiver who, in the end, only has her or his best interest at heart. Family caregivers accept their newfound role, which they fully embrace, in many cases, in an all-consuming manner. They believe that caregiving in dementia is preferably undertaken in the home, where they find themselves, for the most part, reacting to continuously changing, taxing circumstances that progressively worsen over time. Family caregivers seek to manage these circumstances by developing a regimen of personally-suited, flexible and innovative strategies and practices. Alongside what may be considered a more 'organic' approach to caregiving in dementia, family caregivers, nevertheless, lament the solitary nature of the caregiving endeavour. Acceptance through normalisation of their situation allows many to maintain a high level of commitment to their caregiving role, despite their sense of isolation from society.

Sentence level structural analysis

Analysis of the sentence level linguistic and semantic features of the life stories under study reveals the following salient themes and subthemes pertaining to the family caregiver experience of dementia (Table 5.1). They are discussed and illustrated in the sections that follow.

Dementia causes loss

While notions of loss in family caregiving in mental illness centred on material concerns for families and the disruption of expected futures for caregiver and ill family member alike, in the dementia stories under study notions of loss tend to coalesce around the ill family member. As a progressive, degenerative disorder from which there is no hope of recovery, it is unsurprising that the continuing decline experienced by the person with dementia – losses in cognition, bodily function, emotional expression, communication, ability to work and self-awareness amongst others – remain at the forefront of the family caregiver's account (Hinton and Levkoff 1999). The 'extreme' lexicon and material metaphor of natural disaster employed to recount the impact of mental illness on caregivers and their families in the life stories analysed in Chapter 3 are, for the most part, absent from the dementia counterparts. It seems that the disruptions to projected life pathways as well as to the ability to fulfil culturally prescribed familial and social responsibilities are considered to be less traumatic where the ill person is already retired and viewed to be in the latter years of her or his life. The 'battle' metaphor characterising the mental illness corpora is also not drawn

Life stories of family caregiving in dementia　81

Table 5.1 Salient themes and subthemes in Hong Kong Chinese family caregiver stories of dementia

Theme	Subtheme
Dementia causes loss	Progressive decline Embodied (past) versus disembodied (present) identities Role reversal
Obligation to care	Caregiving in the home Caregiving entails management of circumstances Caregiving is solitary Caregiving is burdensome Fear of potential hurdles to optimal caregiving
Acceptance	Value of acceptance and normalisation of circumstances
Explanatory models of dementia	Dementia has a physiological aetiology Dementia has a psychosocial aetiology Dementia has a biogenetic aetiology

on, with two of the three key elements required for effective expression of such a metaphor missing in the illness stories under study in the current chapter (Hawkins 1999. See Chapter 1), namely, a strong alliance with health professionals, family caregiving in dementia being a predominantly solitary, home-based endeavour; and the availability of effective pharmacotherapeutic weapons, which are few and far between in dementia (Qiu 2007).

Uncle Leung has been ill for ten years and his situation gets worse every day. In the initial stage of the disease, Uncle Leung could take care of simple things himself, like taking a bath, but in the latter stage he needed the assistance of others. When thirsty, Uncle Leung could not distinguish between fresh and boiled water, and frequently even drank water from the toilet bowl. Early on Uncle Leung liked to talk, but as time went by he no longer wished to talk. Leung Chi Ming recalls that in the latter stage Uncle Leung could only produce the sound 'nah, nah, nah'. No one knew what he was saying.
[梁伯患病十年, 情況是一天比一天壞. 簡單如洗澡, 病發初期, 梁伯還是會自己來的. 後期就要別人協助. 口乾喝水, 梁伯生熟水不分, 甚至常常喝馬桶內的廁所水. 開始時, 梁伯還喜歡說話. 日子久了, 連話也不大想說. 梁志明記得, 到後期只會發出「哪、哪、哪」的聲音, 沒有人知道他在說什麼.]
(Text 3, HKADAPG 2002, 26–27)

There are two rooms in the three hundred or so square-foot apartment, in one of which lies Wong Yee's mother, more than 80 years of age, a feeding tube in place and her eyes closed. Even though two pillows are used to support her as she sleeps, her head still limply leans to one side …. The mother's situation only gets worse day by day.

[三百多呎的單位內，有兩個房間，其中一個躺著王儀的媽媽，八十多歲，插著喉管，眼睛閉者，縱使用兩個枕頭墊高的睡著，她的頭還是無力的側在一邊 … 媽媽的情況只有一天比一天差.]

(Text 5, HKADAPG 2002, 36–37)

Shuk Yee's condition was, at times, good and, at other times, bad. Watching her ability to deal with some simple things in life gradually deteriorate, progressing from experiencing a little difficulty to being unable to take care of herself, was most difficult to accept.

[淑儀病情時好時壞. 看著她在處理生活上的一些簡單事情的能力逐漸退步，由有點困難發展至無法自我照顧，是最難接受的.]

(Lee 2005, 19)

The attention given to the losses experienced by the ill family member commonly leads to the person being ascribed two identities in the life stories under study: the healthy, embodied person from before the onset of illness and the ill, disembodied person currently being cared for. While characterising any illness experience, the phenomenon is particularly distinctive in the life stories under study with the absence of any hope of the embodied person returning. The impairment that dementia causes to what are commonly viewed as the core elements to a person's identity, that is, cognition, communication, emotion and self-awareness (Hydén and Örulv 2009; Roy 2009; Wiltshire 2000), leads to the identity of the person in illness being devalued in the stories. Much is said about the person in illness in the stories, yet it seems that the 'true' identity of this person remains located in the healthy individual of bygone times. Only through family caregiver recollections of the individual's past life as a talented and supportive parent or spouse can one come to fully know the value of the person now being cared for.

These memories are selectively retained (Garro 2001). In Lee's (2005, 77) autobiography, for example, memory of his wife's choral talent prior to falling ill, which also brings to mind his past acts of thoughtlessness and inconsideration, is subsequently relinquished: 'What is lost is forever lost' [失去了的也永遠失去了]. Roy (2009) points out that such selectivity in recollection can leave the 'truth value' of a family caregiver account of dementia as unreliable as that proffered by the person with dementia (see Chapter 1).

In the eyes of Mrs Luk, her husband was a hardworking and reliable person, so at a very young age she entrusted her own happiness to him. At that time, of course, she could not have reckoned that, today, that strong pair of hands would come to be clutching tightly at her clothing all day long …. 'He was my first boyfriend. He possessed a great sense of responsibility and commitment. And he was of good moral character …. Starting from '95 or

'96 my husband's temperament suddenly changed, becoming very odd. It was difficult for one to accept.'
[在陸太的心目中, 丈夫是一個勤懇可靠的人, 所以年紀輕輕就將自己的幸福交託給他. 當時的她當然估不到那雙強而有力的手, 到今日會變得整天拉著自己的衣衫不放 … 「他是我第一個男友, 很有責任心, 有承擔, 人品又好 … 丈夫在九五、九六年開始, 突然間脾氣變得很古怪, 令人難以接受.」]

(Text 4, HKADAPG 2002, 30–31)

There are two photographs sitting on the sideboard. One is of Ah Kuen's other brothers and sisters; the other is of her mother's life many years ago. At that time she was slightly overweight, but now she is half the size. Ah Kuen's memory of her mother is one of a good wife and loving mother. She didn't like to swear or curse. Previously Mother would also go out for dim sum. A few months ago she could still say a word or two, albeit with much trouble. In recent months she can no longer even speak one or two words.
[組合櫃上, 放了兩幅相片. 一張是亞娟其他兄弟姐妹. 另一張是多年前媽媽的生活照. 那時她略肥胖, 眼前的她, 卻瘦了一半. 亞娟記憶中的媽媽, 是賢妻良母型, 不愛罵人. 以前媽媽也會行街飲茶. 幾個月前, 她還能很辛苦地吐出一、兩個字. 近個月, 連一、兩個字也不會再說了.]

(Text 9, HKADAPG 2002, 70)

No matter what, we lived together like this for more than 40 years. Today I still admire Shuk Yee's amiable and taciturn temperament. It's just a pity that, with the passing of time, she speaks so much less and even no longer speaks at all.[6]
[無論如何, 我們就是這樣共同生活了四十多年. 今天, 我還是欣賞淑儀的隨和、寡言的性格, 只可惜隨著時間的過去, 她說得更少, 甚至不說話了.]

(Lee 2005, 38)

Being viewed as a disembodied subject somewhat devalued by his or her illness (Hydén and Örulv 2009; Roy 2009; Traphagan 2000; Wiltshire 2000) locates the person with dementia in a more passive role, subject to the well-intentioned and benevolent actions of the family caregiver. In many instances, this, in turn, places the caregiver in a role seen previously to belong to the ill family member. The family caregiver's identity, thus, comes to be framed in terms of one formerly ascribed to the person now being cared for: dutiful and dedicated mother, father, wife or husband. In the life stores under study, this identity typically reflects culturally prescribed gendered norms for the adopted role.

Mrs Ng passively fell ill. Ng Bing keeps watch by his wife's side, actively helping her to fight her illness. In reality, one cannot plainly say whose life is being led, when all is said and done.
[吳太是被動地生病, 吳炳守在太太身旁, 主動地協助她抗病. 過得, 到底是誰人的生活, 實在說不清楚.]

(Text 1, HKADAPG 2002, 6)

'Previously, I was a heavily dependent woman …. Now it's turned on its head …. Before I followed him, now he follows me.'
[「我以前是一個依賴性很重的女人 … 現在倒過來 … 以前我跟着他, 現在他跟着我.」]

(Text 4, HKADAPG 2002, 31–32)

I have already reached retirement age and am seven years older than Shuk Yee. I originally thought that Shuk Yee, being younger than I am, could take care of me when I got old. Who would have thought … Shuk Yee is totally dependent on me to live.
[我已到退休年齡, 比淑儀大七年. 原以為淑儀比我年青, 可在我年老時照顧我. 豈料 … 淑儀完全依賴我生活.]

(Lee 2005, 17, 19)

Obligation to care

As with the family caregiver stories of mental illness, there is a strong sense of obligation to care for the ill family member in the dementia counterparts. While hospitalisation, even temporary placement therein, is commonly acknowledged to be necessary in the mental illness stories, in the dementia counterparts the place for giving care is seen to be principally in the home. Episodes of hospitalisation, for example, following falls or in acute infections, are frequently recounted in highly negative terms, while placing ill family members in residential facilities for the aged is commonly resisted, despite acknowledgment of their availability.

Even though her mother has already forgotten who she is and the situation is worsening day by day, she still lives on, in tears, tightly clasping her mother's hand. Everything is like this as a matter of course. Every hardship and burden remains insubstantial …. The doctor said that Mrs Lee's condition cannot drag on, that she must be admitted to hospital so that someone can take care of her around the clock. Objectively speaking, this recommendation, without a doubt, is a good thing for hardworking Ah Mei and the in-need-of-care Mrs Lee, yet Ah Mei is wholly unwilling to do it. 'How could I be willing to send Mother into hospital? We have always relied on each other for survival.'
[縱然媽媽已忘記她是誰, 情況亦一天比一天壞, 她仍然是含著淚水, 緊緊拉著媽媽的手活下去. 一切都是那麼的理所當然, 一切的困苦、負擔, 都是沒重量 … 醫生說李婆婆的病情已不能拖, 一定要入醫院, 好讓有人可以全天候的照顧她. 客觀來說, 這個建議, 無疑對於要為口奔馳的阿美, 及需要人照顧的李婆婆來說, 是一件好事, 但是阿美卻有一千一萬個不捨得. 「我怎會捨得送媽媽進醫院? 我們一直相依為命.」]

(Text 6, HKADAPG 2002, 42, 44)

Several months ago, a placement at a home for the elderly, for which Mr Hung had been waiting a long time, finally became available. Hung Ling and her brothers decided not to let their father move in, because he can rely on them as a family, along with the home-help, to still be able to take care of him.

[幾個月前, 洪爸爸輪候多時的老人院終於輪到, 洪玲、哥哥及弟弟決定不讓爸爸搬進去, 因為憑他們一家人, 再加上工人尚有能力照顧他.]

(Text 8, HKADAPG 2002, 62)

Home, it need not be luxurious but must be cosy and graceful, ... is precisely a part of our two-person world .... When we go for a walk outside, we can take in all the open air, not like staying in a hospital or a home for the elderly, waiting for the nigh-on end of one's life.

[家, 毋需豪華, 但一定要舒適清雅, ... 便是屬於我倆的二人世界 ... 在外面走動, 能吸收大量自由的空氣, 不像住在醫院、老人院裡般等待大限來臨.]

(Lee 2005, 52–53)

In the life stories under study, the act of family caregiving is characterised principally by the management of circumstances faced by the caregiver. Given that caregiving takes place in the home and that the ill family member's condition is progressively deteriorating, it is probably unsurprising that the life stories devote a significant amount of attention to recounting the practical responses to problematic issues and events that arise in day-to-day life. The acts of maintaining a functional home life and, wherever possible, a semblance of a social life that includes the ill family member, seemingly, serve as immediate motivating forces for caregiving, sustained in the longer term by the family caregiver's sense of filial duty. Unlike the family caregiver stories in mental illness, family caregiver actions in the dementia counterparts tend to be more concerned with attenuating or moderating challenging circumstances to suit the parties in question, namely, the caregiver and the ill family member. Family caregivers tend to react spontaneously and intuitively as these circumstances arise. They do not appear to be driven, as many family caregivers in the mental illness stories were, to demonstrate absolute control over their circumstances, both current and future, in order to meet cultural expectations to resolutely give care and return the ill family member to a productive role in society, for example, by enforcing medication compliance.

Seeing Ng Bing's new homemade invention I think that Mrs Ng has been really blessed in her illness. Ng Bing, himself, is already 80 years of age, yet still is so thoughtful in his consideration for her. Without time to open my mouth in praise of him, Ng Bing excitedly drags me over to see an even more recent invention, namely, a homemade commode close to the bed. The lid of the commode had been purchased. Handwritten on it were the two Chinese characters for 'toilet' .... Because Mrs Ng had once taken a fall going to the toilet, Ng Bing had made for her this toilet placed beside the bed, so as to allow her to go to the toilet with ease.

[看著吳炳的土製新發明, 覺得吳太病得真幸福, 吳炳自己都八十歲了, 還替她設想得那麼周到. 來不及開口讚美他, 吳炳又興緻勃勃拉我去看一個更

新的發明, 那是一個離睡床不遠的自製馬桶, 馬桶蓋是買回來的, 手寫廁所
兩個字 … 因為吳太上廁所跌過一跤, 吳炳就替她造出這個放在床邊的廁
所, 好讓她就近如廁.]

(Text 1, HKADAPG 2002, 3)

Apart from furniture, nothing can be seen. The glass cabinet in the
sideboard is also empty. A big black box is built onto the back of the
television, hiding any power cables and plugs. The clock and the spirit tablet
hang close to the ceiling. Locks are installed on everything. The telephone is
also locked inside a wooden box. This is all to prevent Mrs Law touching
them …. Just like a child, 68-year-old Mrs Law is too fond of playing. Once
she sees something she is 'all hands'. As a result, Mr Law can only deal with
problems as they present themselves.
[除了傢俬外, 甚麼也看不到, 組合櫃的玻璃內也是空的. 電視背上蓋了個
大黑盒, 看不到任何電線插蘇. 大鐘和神位, 掛到接近天花板. 所有東西
都裝了鎖, 電話也鎖在木箱內. 這全都是為了避免羅太摸到 … 六十八歲的
羅太, 像小孩子一樣貪玩, 見到甚麼都會「手多多.」 於是羅先生唯有見招
拆招.]

(Text 7, HKADAPG 2002, 50–51)

Through the centre's day care service, I was given some time and space for
myself …. After steadying my own mind, then I was able to plan and make
full use of the time set aside.
[通過了中心的日間護理服務, 讓我有自己的時間空間 … 當我穩定自己的心
理後, 便能計劃並充分利用騰出來的時間.]

(Lee 2005, 33)

Family caregiving in dementia is a more solitary endeavour in the life stories
under study than in their mental illness counterparts. As in the mental illness
counterparts, the task of caregiving commonly falls upon the shoulders of one
family member, usually the spouse or daughter. Yet, unlike the mental illness
counterparts, support for this person in the family caregiving role, from health
professionals, caregivers in like circumstances, other family members or society
more broadly, is less evident in the stories. Some people make use of day care
placements, yet, for the most part, they single-handedly carry out caregiving
duties in the home setting, the primary location of caregiving.

'My older brother said, "My wife is not able to take care of Mother, you
know. You [his sister and the mother with dementia] go find a place for
yourselves to move into." Since then, I have taken care of Mother on my
own. Most of the time each day, apart from work and sleep, is spent
together with Mother.'
[「哥哥說:『我太太不會照顧媽媽的啦, 你們自己找地方搬吧.』自此, 我便獨
立照顧媽媽, 每天最多的時間, 除了工作及睡覺, 便是跟媽媽在一起.」]

(Text 6, HKADAPG 2002, 44)

The brothers and younger sister who Mother loved rather dearly each had their own families. It was quite difficult for them to take her in. The responsibility for taking care of Mother quite naturally fell onto Ah Kuen, who was living by herself.

[媽媽比較疼愛的兄弟妹妹都各自有自己的家庭，很難接受她．照顧母親的責任，很自然地落在獨自一人住的亞娟身上．]

(Text 9, HKADAPG 2002, 67)

Thinking of me having tirelessly worked hard all of my life, being a member of the middle class and having reached the required retirement age, yet unable to gain the attention of society. I felt really isolated and helpless. Even though I loudly cried out for 'help', nobody was able to hear.

[想到自己一生努力工作不懈，作為中產階級，到了有需要的退休年齡，卻得不到社會的照顧，實在是孤立無助，即使大呼「救命」也沒有人能聽到．]

(Lee 2005, 32)

Being obliged to give care to a loved one with an incurable illness, frequently alone in the home, and having to respond to the increasingly challenging circumstances that progressively emerge over time, cause family caregiving to be recounted in the life stories under study as a particularly burdensome experience. That family caregiving in dementia is burdensome is, of course, well documented across many cultural settings (Bartlett *et al.* 1993; Biegel *et al.* 1991; Lai 2007; Li and Lemke 2004; Petrus and Wing-chung 2005). Yet, despite the burden, a commitment to resolutely give care features throughout the corpus under study.

The heavy demands and personal restrictions that attend family caregiving in dementia, however, do lead some to contemplate abandoning the family caregiving responsibility (Mackenzie and Holroyd 1996). Similar thoughts were also entertained in the mental illness corpus and, at times, were carried through (see Chapter 3). Also reminiscent of the mental illness corpus, rare episodes of violence, in this case limited to actions by the ill family member and not by the family caregiver, prove particularly detrimental to motivation and perseverance in the caregiving role.

Uncle Leung would also often get angry. When he felt that people didn't understand him, he would also have the tendency to be violent and hit people. 'To be honest, during the period of taking care of Father, sometimes I also felt pressured. I felt that I might not be able to take care of him for a long period of time, so I also applied for Father to go into a residential home for the elderly', Leung Chi Ming said.

[梁伯發脾氣也是常有的事，覺得人家不明白他時，還會有打人的暴力傾向．「坦白說，照顧父親期間，有時也感到壓力，覺得自己或許不能長久照顧他，所以也有替父親申請入住老人院舍．」 梁志明說．]

(Text 3, HKADAPG 2002, 27)

'At that time I didn't know what Alzheimer's disease was at all. I only saw her [mother's] bad temper. She would swear at people and hit people for no reason at all. She would beat them fiercely. If you weren't careful you'd get scratched.' …. More than six years has past and Ah Kuen is exhausted beyond description. What she feels most is: she has no freedom at all, cut off from the outside world. During this time she has, on occasion, thought of giving up.

[「那時根本不知道甚麼是老年痴呆症，只見她脾氣不好，會無緣無故罵人打人，打得很大力，一不小心會被抓傷。」… 六年多來，亞娟辛苦得不知如何形容，最大的感覺是: 甚麼自由也沒有，與外間斷絕. 期間曾經想過放棄.]

(Text 9, HKADAPG 2002, 68, 71)

Because she could get lost, one had to take special care when doing outdoor activities. Going to a public toilet also became a big problem. What's more, early on she experienced hallucinations or would keep staring at other people. So in public places one also encountered a lot of difficulties and embarrassment …. In a family, is it right that complete responsibility for caregiving is taken on by one person? Why can't she be placed in the hands of a professional caregiver, so I can freely enjoy a world of my own?

[由於她會迷路，到外面活動要特別小心，而去公共洗手間也成了一個大問題. 加上早期她有幻覺，又或不斷地凝望別人，所以在公共場所裡也遇到不少困難和尷尬情況 … 一個家庭裡, 由一個人完全承擔照顧責任是對的嗎? 為甚麼不可以把她放在專業的照顧者手中，讓我可以享受海闊天空的個人世界?]

(Lee 2005, 19, 93)

Others remain fully committed in the stories in question to the family caregiving endeavour, but fear that they may not be able to maintain their roles with distinction over the longer term. They do not question their competence as family caregivers, as some did in the mental illness counterparts (see Chapter 3). Thus, self-blame is not commonly expressed. Fear, however, is expressed over the ability to continue to give care in the home, when the continuing health and availability of the family caregiver cannot be assured.

Mentally, Yeung Chu Fang still hides a concern that cannot be spoken about. 'At the moment I am still able to take care of him. But what about in the future? If I, myself, also fall ill, what's to be done with him?'

[心理上, 楊楚芳還是隱隱然有說不出的憂慮. 「現在我還有能力照顧他. 將來呢? 要是我自己也生病, 他怎麼辦呢?」]

(Text 2, HKADAPG 2002, 19)

'Sometimes I would think, if, one day, I were to die before him, then what would happen? He probably would be sent to a home for the elderly.' …. Mrs Luk blandly speaks these few sentences. Yet, on hearing them, the bystander feels that there is a hint of sadness and poignancy which cannot be put into words.

[「有時候, 我都會想, 一旦有一天, 我比他早去世, 那又會如何呢? 可能他會被送進老人院.」 ... 陸太淡淡的說出這幾句話, 旁人聽進耳中, 卻覺得有一種說不出的辛酸及蕩氣迴腸的味道.]

(Text 4, HKADAPG 2002, 33–34)

If I'm under tremendous pressure for a long period, might I also become another dementia sufferer? And if I fall ill, how am I to take care of another sick person?
[長期承受沉重的壓力, 我也會變成另一個痴呆病者? 如果我病了, 又怎樣照顧另一個病人呢?]

(Lee 2005, 91–92)

Acceptance

Many of the life stories emphasise the importance of acceptance of the illness and the attendant position that family caregivers find themselves in. While the mental illness stories tended to promote a proactive response to remedy and overcome the tragedy that had befallen the ill family member, the end-goal being successfully returning the ill family member to society, many of the dementia counterparts recommend acknowledging the reality of the circumstances that family caregivers finds themselves in and envisioning these circumstances as part of the natural course of life. Religion plays a role in reaching acceptance, for some.

Living to 80 years of age, one certainly is entitled to sum up life. Ng Bing says: 'Such is life, you know. Before 80 years of age it was quite easy. At 81 years of age it started to get complicated. I very much take things philosophically; I deal with things one step at a time. If things are going smoothly, then I travel a little happier; if things are hard to pass, then I slowly think of a plan.'
[活到八十歲, 當然有資格總結人生, 吳炳說:「人生就是這樣喇. 八十歲前還好端端, 到八十一歲就開始複雜. 我好達觀, 見步行步, 順利的話, 就行得歡愉點; 難行的話, 就慢慢諗囉.」]

(Text 1, HKADAPG 2002, 10)

Early on, Hong Ling didn't eat or sleep well. She was always thinking about how she could help her father and was liable to end up in a dead end. Afterward, she slowly let go a little, 'Every single thing also has its law of behaviour; let nature take its course.' Previously, reading the Buddhist scriptures made one a little balanced and at peace. Now, she can apply and integrate this into her daily life.
[初期, 洪玲食不好睡不安, 總是想著如何可以幫到爸爸, 容易鑽牛角尖. 後來, 她慢慢的放開一點, 「每一樣東西也有其規律, 順其自然.」 以前讀佛經令人祥和一點. 現在, 她可以應用及融匯在日常生活中.]

(Text 8, HKADAPG 2002, 61)

I eventually recognised the existing reality and actively thought about how to accept and cope with it …. In fact, Shuk Yee can be considered to not be suffering from any serious illness, it's just that the signs of ageing have appeared comparatively early in life. Sometimes I even feel that Shuk Yee is abominable and adorable like a child …. In the most difficult times, I seek to pray. I pour out my predicament to God and long for Him to be able to grant me strength.

[我終於認識到現實之存在而積極地思考如何去接受和應付 … 其實淑儀也不算是患了甚麼大病, 只是人生的老化現象出現得較早; 有時候, 我會覺得淑儀像小孩子般可惡和可愛 … 在最困難時, 我嘗試祈禱, 向神傾吐我的困境, 並且憧憬著祂能賜我力量.]

(Lee 2005, 20, 30)

Explanatory models of dementia

Only three stories explicitly make reference to the aetiological basis of the family member's illness, outside of normative decline in old age. One story links dementia to a cardiovascular disorder that the family member suffers from. Another story links the illness to psychosocial stress that the family member had experienced in being the subject of criticism during the Cultural Revolution and in being separated from her family for many years, in neighbouring mainland China. The third story makes reference to a biogenetic aetiology in noting a history of similar illness in the ill spouse's family.

All in all, for most of the family caregivers the aetiological basis to dementia remains of little consequence. Biological and environmental explanations are entertained only on occasion and, where done so, there is no consistency across the stories in question in the explanation volunteered. What is more, despite recurring family caregiver accounts (in the life stories under study) of regular contact with health services, the biomedical explanatory model is not readily embraced across the family caregiver corpus.

'Ordinary people, of course, do not understand what Alzheimer's disease is. I just hear people say that it might be an effect brought about by medication used to treat the heart.' But Mr Law thinks that it might be because there's always been a problem with Mrs Law's blood.

[「普通人當然不明白甚麼是老年痴呆症, 只聽人說, 可能是因為醫心臟的藥造成的影響.」 但羅先生卻認為, 可能是因為羅太的血一直有問題.]

(Text 7, HKADAPG 2002, 54)

Her father had taken the other children to Hong Kong long before the Cultural Revolution. Her mother and another two younger sisters did not get approval and stayed in Guangzhou. Then came the public criticism and denunciation: from time to time someone would knock on the door in the middle of the night and call on her mother to attend a 'meeting'. Sometimes she would be gone for several days while the younger sisters had no food to eat. Her mother was on the verge of killing herself .... Her mother and younger sisters moved to Shenzhen. Later on, the younger sisters got married and she lived alone for seven years in Shenzhen where she probably entertained foolish ideas way too often. She became quite uncertain .... Ah Kuen thinks that her mother's illness had probably already been lurking in Shenzhen, only nobody was aware of it.

[文革前, 爸爸早已帶著其他孩子來到香港, 媽媽和另外兩個妹妹不獲批准, 留在廣州. 然後, 批鬥來了: 半夜不時有人來敲門, 叫媽媽去「開會」, 有時一去幾天, 妹妹便沒有飯吃. 媽媽差點自殺死了 … 媽媽與妹妹搬到深圳, 後來妹妹結婚, 她就一個人住在深圳七年, 可能胡思亂想得太多, 人變得很飄忽 … 亞娟想, 媽媽的病可能在深圳時已潛伏, 只是沒有人知道.]

(Text 9, HKADAPG 2002, 66)

The doctor suggested that this kind of illness might be hereditary .... I vaguely remembered … a close relative of Shuk Yee, who we all called 'Third Great Aunt' .... She … appeared a little bit like Shuk Yee in her current state .... I tried to ask my mother-in-law for information about Third Great Aunt, but she was always unable to give me a satisfactory answer. I raised the seriousness of hereditary illness to future generations … but she strongly denied that Third Great Aunt was immediate family and categorically denied that Third Great Aunt was suffering from Alzheimer's disease .... I cannot tell whether I worry too much about [such] matters, but I truly don't want my manuscript to have a sequel in the future.

[醫生提出了這種病可能是遺傳性的 … 依稀記得 … 一位淑儀的親人, 我們都稱呼她為「三大姑母」 … 她 … 有點像淑儀現時的情況 … 我嘗試追問外母關於三大姑母的資料, 她總不能給我滿意的答覆. 我提出遺傳病對後代的嚴重性 … 只是極力否認三大姑母是直系親屬, 也斷言否認三大姑母患的是老人痴呆病 … 我不能分辨我對事情是否過於憂慮, 但真不希望將來我的文章還有續集.]

(Lee 2005, 79–81)

Comprehensive understanding

Following the analysis undertaken in Chapter 2, the meanings expressed in people's life stories of family caregiving in dementia are now examined in terms of how they are shaped by culture. This entails consideration of and illustration by means of the temporal and causal ordering of life events, the claiming and refashioning of identities, and language use.

As in mental illness, dementia marks a temporal juncture in the family caregiver's life. This juncture, however, does not equate to the tumultuous 'biographical disruption' experienced by the family caregivers in mental illness (Bury 1982, 169). The language of catastrophe and long-term struggle, which characterised the family caregiver stories of mental illness, remains broadly unvoiced in the dementia counterparts. The larger narrative focus on the impact on the caregiver and family, which characterised the family caregiver stories of mental illness, coalesces more around the ill family member in the dementia counterparts. The normative life pathway and attendant social responsibilities in Chinese culture likely shape the accounts of family caregiving in dementia in this way: first, by prescribing a duty to give care to family members in old age, dementia usually manifesting in a person's latter years; and, second, by conflating the cognitive and physical losses that characterise dementia with normative decline in old age.

Caring for the elderly is deeply-seated in Chinese culture, an expression of filial piety (Cheng 2009; Chow 2001; Chung 2001; Gray *et al.* 2009; Lai 2007, 2010; Laidlaw *et al.* 2010; Lam 2006; Liu, W. *et al.* 2008; Petrus and Wing-chung 2005; Wang *et al.* 2006; Zhan 2006); or fulfilment of the 'inter-generational contract' (Cheung and Kwan 2009, 192), deemed a more appropriate characterisation in the increasingly nuclear familial forms found in contemporary urban Chinese societies (Chow 1990; Holroyd 2001). As a consequence, family members anticipate that such a role will occur at some stage in their lives. The role may be challenging, but it is not unexpected (Ho *et al.* 2003). Thus, in the dementia corpus, the family caregiver's own plight may be viewed as not so remarkable that it deserves to be the focal point of the life stories told. The experience of loss tends to coalesce around the ill family member. Furthermore, the family caregiver's own plight, when recounted, does not warrant the use of the immoderate forms of language that characterised the mental illness counterparts. Likewise, any 'sense of achievement' [成功感] voiced in successful performance of the family caregiving role arouses 'very ambiguous feelings' [心情矛盾極了] (Lee 2005, 113).

Chinese cultural norms prescribe that care for the elderly should take place in the home setting (Cheng 2009; Chow 1990; Holroyd 2001; Lai 2007, 2010; Lam 2006; Liu, W. *et al.*, 2008). This resonates in the dementia stories under study with caregiving primarily being a home-based endeavour. Placement in institutional care is resisted by the family caregivers, as prescribed by cultural norms (Gallagher-Thompson *et al.* 2010; Gray *et al.* 2009; Lam 2006; Leung 2001; Leung and Gallagher-Thompson 2005; Liu, W. *et al.* 2008; Petrus and Wing-chung 2005; Wang *et al.* 2006). The 'fundamental moral challenge' (Hydén 1995, 67) in the life stories under study, therefore, lies in meeting the cultural expectation to provide care in the home. This leads many family caregivers to worry about circumstances that may hinder their ability to maintain home care, such as illness, exhaustion, death or ill family member violence. Some even contemplate permanent institutionalisation, despite the moral transgression this would signify.

In the family caregiver stories of mental illness, the moral challenge entailed caregiving at all costs in order to ensure that the ill family member is protected, not socially disruptive, compliant with therapeutic regimes and nurtured to regain full social functioning. Where this moral challenge was not met, for example, where the ill family member remained acutely symptomatic or where the family caregiving endeavour was abandoned, there was self-admonishment. Family caregivers spoke of themselves as having 'failed' and as being 'incompetent'. In the family caregiver stories of dementia, failure to meet the moral challenge to maintain caregiving in the home, or contemplation of such, is not accompanied by the self-admonishment voiced in the mental illness counterparts. Institutional placement is vehemently resisted by the family caregivers in dementia, as cultural norms prescribe, but some caregivers do contemplate and carry out such action, without apparent self-blame, in the end stage of disease or where there is ongoing violent behaviour by the ill family member. It seems that for some family caregivers there can be 'exoneration' from self-blame when they morally transgress by institutionalising an ill family member with dementia (Bury 2001).

The regional setting may be influential in this. Institutional care for the elderly is tacitly legitimised by government discourse in Hong Kong. Holroyd (2001, 1126) quotes the 1991 'White Paper on *Social Welfare in the 1990s and Beyond*' prepared by the Hong Kong regional government, which states:

> While it will remain our policy to encourage the care of the elderly by the family members within a family context and to strengthen support for their carers, it should also be recognised that the needs of the elderly vary and that residential care for some may be the most appropriate service.

Ho *et al.* (2003, 316) also report in a study of Chinese Canadians that greater access to institutional facilities allows the use of these facilities to be 'normalized' despite a 'strong sense of obligation to care for the elderly ... and the dislike of the notion of institutionalizing'. Awareness of access to aged care facilities in Hong Kong (Cheng 2009), along with a legitimisation of their use in certain circumstances (Cheng 2009; Ho *et al.* 2003), may, for some, moderate the degree of moral transgression attending their use, despite the cultural expectation to give care in the home. This would demonstrate, as Bartlett *et al.* (1993, 412) observe in stories about caregiving in dementia published in the West, 'the complexity of family caregiving and its relation to moral reasoning, and the salience of the social and political context to decisions about care'. Nevertheless, moral reasoning in the Hong Kong Chinese family caregiver stories under study remains heavily shaped by culture in that, in most of the life stories, permanent institutionalisation is only ever contemplated by the family caregivers; it is never actually carried out.

The second way culture shapes many of the life stories under study, in ways that likely militate against the framing of the family caregiving experience in dementia as a tumultuous 'biographical disruption' (Bury 1982, 169), is by conflating the cognitive and physical losses experienced in dementia with normative decline in old age. In Chinese culture, physical and cognitive decline normally accompany old age. As such, the physical and cognitive decline experienced in dementia is readily equated to normative old age (Gray *et al.* 2009; Hicks and Lam 1999; Ikels 2002; Lai and Surood 2009; Liu, D. *et al.* 2008; Wang *et al.* 2006). Hinton *et al.* (2000, 125) claim that this ambiguity between the pathology of dementia and the normal process of ageing in

Chinese culture can be traced 'to traditional Chinese views of the life course as a cyclical process consisting of four phases, the last phase characterized by return to a childlike state.' Thus, in the life stories under study, attention is drawn to the ill family members, who are often ascribed the qualities of a child [像小孩子一樣]. The dominant metaphor in the family caregiving in dementia stories, therefore, does not locate the ill family member in the midst of a battle or a natural disaster, as in the mental illness counterparts, but in the innocence and mischievousness of childhood. Such language harks back to the normal life cycle in Chinese culture and absolves the person, and their family, from blame (Hinton and Levkoff 1999).

Normalising the signs of dementia and palliating them by way of the 'child' metaphor ward off the stigma that attends any admission of degenerative illness in Chinese culture (Hinton and Levkoff 1999). Face is preserved where responsibility for the condition resides in the normal cycle of life (Hinton *et al.* 2000). Nevertheless, Liu *et al.* (2008, 293) report that Chinese Americans do make 'clear distinctions between older persons who had "aged well" and those who had aged less well …. People with dementia … fall[ing] into the latter category.' Traphagan (2000) documents a similar phenomenon in rural-dwelling Japanese, the basis of which is traceable to Japan's Confucian-heritage culture. Moreover, Liu, D. *et al.* (2008, 296) find in their study of Chinese Americans that 'when applied to people with dementia, this negative but "normalized" trajectory of ageing carried with it a soft stigma that was distinct from that of chronic and severe mental illness.' This softer form of stigma remains 'shaped by powerful cultural constructs' that are sufficient to cause a 'tangible fading of social network' in family caregiving in dementia (Liu, D. *et al.* 2008, 296. See also Mackenzie and Holroyd, 1996). In the life stories under study, this may have contributed to the solitude frequently spoken of by family caregivers. All the same, the more extreme displays of 'felt stigma' (Scambler 2004, 33) that characterised the family caregiver stories of mental illness, with accounts of careful concealment of the illness from family members and unsuspecting health professionals, do not feature in the dementia counterparts.

Cohen (1998, 33) states that 'Senility is acutely attributional: it almost always requires two bodies, a senile body and a secondary body', usually the family caregiver, 'that recognizes a change in the first.' In the life stories under study, family caregivers engage both the notion of present loss and productive past in constructing the subjectivity of the family member they now care for. The onset of illness-related decline constitutes the temporal marker of the person 'of now' (disembodied) and the person 'from before' (embodied) (Cohen 1998; Hinton and Levkoff 1999; Roy 2009; Traphagan 2000; Wiltshire 2000). Yet both identities, embodied and disembodied, remain contemporaneous in the family caregiver stories. It seems that in the eyes of the family caregiver, the person being cared for is, at once, the person from before and the person of now. The losses that befall the person with dementia are very real and so subject to a great deal of attention in the family caregiver stories; more attention, in fact, than is given to the family caregivers' own plight (see above). Description of these losses, however, also brings to mind the value and richness of the person from before, accounts of which permeate the family caregiver stories to such an extent that the embodied person from before becomes as tangible an identity in the present as the now disembodied person in illness. The two identities coexist contemporaneously, reconciling what constitute contrasting 'beings' of the person being cared for: one valued and celebrated; one devalued and mourned (Hinton and Levkoff 1999). As a consequence, in the life stories under study, the person with dementia, in the end, rarely constitutes an object of pity or aversion. The disembodied identity is seemingly assuaged by the embodied identity that continues to be, maintaining the sense of personhood of the family member being cared for, while, necessarily, diminishing the value of this person in illness (Liu *et al.* 2008).

Holroyd (2001, 1132) sees this reviving of the embodied identity of the person being cared for as motivated by the Chinese cultural value of 'reciprocity'. In studies conducted in mainland China (Holroyd 2003; Holroyd and Mackenzie 1997) and Hong Kong (Holroyd 2001, 2003), caring for elderly family members with chronic ailments is found to be characterised by 'family member attempts to draw on previous memories to sustain caregiving as an act of love or sentiment', with 'these memories juxtapose[d] with the reality of the current situation altered by physical and mental decline' (Holroyd and Mackenzie 1997, 359). In so doing, family caregivers are seen to be 'justify[ing] the rendering of the current care' in terms of 'duty in return for past acts' (Holroyd and Mackenzie 1997, 360). Engaging the cultural value of reciprocity in caring for the elderly, it seems, is contingent on the Chinese family caregiver's capacity to revive positive memories of the embodied person from before. Analysis of the life stories in the current chapter suggests that this is also true in caring for family members with dementia, at least where the revived memory of the embodied person from before does not, at the same time, call to mind past misdeeds by the family caregiver.

In the life stories under study, the embodied identity of the person from before is also appropriated by some family members as they reformulate their own identities in their newfound role as caregiver. Wives take on roles seen previously to be held by their now ill husbands (and vice versa); children take on roles seen previously to be held by their now ill mothers or fathers. Echoing what Wiltshire (2000, 415) observes in stories of dementia told in the West, 'the balance ... between carer and patient is upset' with 'a kind of devolution of one selfhood into another.' In the life stories under study, the identity appropriated from the family member now being cared for reflects a romanticised and gendered conception of that person's role in the family before the onset of illness. Mothers and wives are remembered as kind, supportive, caring and dedicated. Fathers and husbands are remembered as strong, hardworking, dependable and breadwinning. This reflects, as Tebbe (2008) observes, the centrality of 'idealized and sanitized' (212) memories of past family life in a person's 'quest for self-definition' (201). In the case of the life stories under study, goodness and integrity are measured by a person's dutiful compliance with culturally prescribed gender norms.

Holroyd (2001, 1132), in a study of Chinese daughters caring for elderly parents in Hong Kong, finds that many actually appropriate the disembodied identity of the person being cared for:

> Daughters, by caring for their parents' bodies – bodies with ever-changing margins – come to have many similar characteristics. This was manifest most visibly when daughters became ill or claimed to 'feel not quite themselves' as a result of endless and repetitive caregiving.

In like manner, a husband caring for his wife with dementia in one of the life stories under study also fears, for a moment, as cited in the preceding analysis, 'If I'm under tremendous pressure for a long period, might I also become another dementia sufferer?' [長期承受沉重的壓力, 我也會變成另一個痴呆患者?] (Lee 2005, 91). This, of course, is contemplative, and elsewhere in the life story the husband appropriates his wife's embodied identity from before.

Thus, memory of the value and richness of the embodied person from before as well as appropriation of her or his embodied identity – albeit selective, romanticised and gendered – maintain a resonance in the present of the person from before. This meets an essential condition for the expression of the Chinese cultural value of reciprocity. This also provides a reassuring thread of continuity between the family caregiver's past and present lives (Charon 2006), similar to that found in the life stories of family caregiving in mental illness analysed in Chapter 3, where people looked to their own pasts, for example, childrearing, to reconcile their current roles as family caregivers in mental illness. Nevertheless, directing the positive attributes to the embodied person from before also unavoidably devalues the (disembodied) person of the present.

Similar to the personal stories of mental illness, the life stories under study shy away from a biomedical aetiological explanation for the family member's illness-related decline. This occurs despite the fact that ongoing medical intervention, principally by means of hospital out-patient services, is acknowledged in most of the life stories. Family caregivers more commonly ascribe the family member's illness-related decline to normative ageing, as noted earlier. Their life stories, therefore, contrast with those of the family caregivers in mental illness where the cause for the family member's disembodiment and problematic behaviours is commonly located in the pathophysiology of illness. Such an aetiological explanation also characterises family caregiving in dementia in the West (Gray *et al.* 2009).

It seems that, similar to the people with a mental illness whose life stories were analysed in Chapter 2, the family caregivers in the life stories under study may feel that a biomedical aetiological explanation can attract the 'hard' stigma that attends any public admission of degenerative illness, such as dementia, in Chinese culture (Gray *et al.* 2009; Hinton *et al.* 2000; Jones *et al.* 2006). This was less of a threat for the family caregivers in mental illness whose life stories were analysed in Chapter 3, because they are one step removed from the illness, in not being a sufferer, and the readers of their stories were likely to be knowledgeable and sympathetic family caregivers who have lived similar experiences (a support group of fellow family caregivers in mental illness). The testimonies proffered in the life stories under study, however, are directed toward a general public who may have little understanding of family caregiving in dementia and who may hold views highly informed by cultural stigma. 'Felt stigma' (Scambler 2004) likely becomes more of an issue when the readers of a life story are not informed and sympathetic insiders, thus silencing allusions to the biomedical aetiological explanation in the life stories under study.

Where a biogenetic basis to dementia is voiced in one life story in the dementia corpus, Lee's (2005) story, the 'hard' form of cultural stigma unmistakeably surfaces. In the story, the denial by a relative of Lee's ill wife that her great aunt had dementia, when she evidently did, together with the denial that the great aunt was a direct kin, point to a prevailing attitude amongst Chinese people that the presence of such illness in a family equates to, in Lee's (2005, 80) words, 'sin' [罪惡]. In the story, Lee also notes that the Chinese expression for dementia [老人痴呆] was once a commonly used insult [用來罵人的名詞] (Lee 2005, 80). Sontag (1989, 58) states that

> Any important disease whose causality is murky, and for which treatment is ineffectual, tends to be awash in significance …. The disease itself becomes a metaphor …. The disease becomes adjectival … projected onto the world.

The cultural projection in the case of the Chinese expression for dementia appears decidedly 'derogatory' [7] (Liu *et al.* 2008, 295).

Conclusion

Analysis of the Hong Kong Chinese life stories of family caregiving in dementia has documented how culture shapes the temporal and causal ordering of life events, the identities claimed and refashioned, and language use in the stories in question. In contrast to the life stories of family caregiving in mental illness analysed in Chapter 3, culture shapes the cognitive and physical losses that attend dementia in a way that often results in them being normalised, conflated with normative decline in old age. This occurs despite the family caregivers' contact with health professionals reported in the stories. Cultural stigma likely militates against invoking a biomedical aetiology to explain the family member's decline.

Framing the signs of dementia as normative ageing causes the language employed to describe family caregiving in dementia to be more tempered than that employed to describe family caregiving in mental illness. Caring for elderly family members in the home is an anticipated event in Chinese culture (filiality/inter-generational contract) and so less biographically disruptive. Most notions of disruption and loss in the life stories under study coalesce around the ill family member. These, too, are tempered by figuratively linking the ill family member's circumstances to the innocence and mischievousness of childhood, rather than to the fervour of battle or turmoil of natural calamity.

As in the family caregiver stories of mental illness, people look to the past to reconcile current roles. Yet, in contrast to the mental illness counterparts, people look to memories, not of themselves, but of the person they now care for. Positive memories of the embodied person from before meet an essential condition for expression of the Chinese cultural value of reciprocity (Holroyd 2001, 2003; Holroyd and Mackenzie 1997). Some people also refashion identities in their newfound role as family caregiver through romanticised and gendered memories of the person from before. As such, their 'new selves' continue to look to the past. Looking to the past, also a feature of the life stories of family caregiving in mental illness, establishes a degree of continuity between the caregiver's past and present lives, providing reassurance amidst the challenges now faced (Charon 2006). A consequent cost, however, is borne by the person being cared for, whose (disembodied) personhood of now is necessarily devalued.

In addition to the cultural shaping documented in the current chapter, the unique socio-political context of Hong Kong may also be in evidence. There appears to be moderation in the degree of moral transgression ascribed to permanent institutionalisation of the ill family member. This may stem from the availability of institutional care in Hong Kong and the tacit legitimisation of such care by government discourse. Religion also plays a role for some in achieving acceptance of the circumstances they now face. Religion remains freely practised in Hong Kong following the British departure in 1997, while remaining potentially problematic in mainland China due to the communist government's historical misgivings about religious practice and contemporary concerns about religious sects.

In sum, this chapter's analysis of life stories of family caregiving in dementia complements the analysis of life stories of mental illness undertaken in Chapters 2 and 3. The analysis has identified and considered similarities and differences in how culture shapes the life stories in question. Following the practice of the earlier chapters, the next chapter turns to filmic stories of family caregiving in dementia in order to examine how culture shapes stories told from outside of the experience (Brody 2003; Hydén 1997).

6 Filmic stories of family caregiving in dementia

In this chapter we explore how culture shapes the filmic stories of people caring for a family member with dementia recounted in two contemporary mainland Chinese productions, the film *Gone is the One Who Held Me Dearest in the World* [世界上最疼我的那个人去了] and the television serial drama *Watch for the Happiness* [守望幸福]. As noted in Chapters 1 and 4, filmic stories are generally told from outside of the life experience. Analysis of the filmic stories undertaken in the current chapter, therefore, can usefully complement the analysis of the life stories undertaken in Chapter 5. At the same time, the prevailing meta-narrative that circulates in a cultural community, in this case in relation to family caregiving in dementia, can be more clearly identified. This meta-narrative communicates a culturally dominant view of family caregiving in dementia, aspects of which may have remained hidden from view in the life stories told by those inside the experience.

The two productions under study, *Gone is the One Who Held Me Dearest in the World* and *Watch for the Happiness*, were released in 2002 and 2005, respectively. The plots of both productions centre on the challenges of family life and family relations in contemporary urban mainland China. In both productions, family life and family relations are complicated by the sudden appearance of signs of dementia in an elderly mother. Dementia or, more specifically, family caregiving in dementia, therefore, constitutes a visible subplot in both productions, serving to augment and amplify the productions' primary plot dealing with family life and family relations in contemporary urban mainland China. The visibility of the dementia subplot and the contemporaneity of the productions in question drove their selection for analysis.

Examining family life and family relations for the purpose of social or political critique finds precedence in the Chinese literary tradition. Most notable are the literary classics *Dream of the Red Chamber* [红楼梦], written by Cao Xueqin [曹雪芹] in the eighteenth century, and *The Family* [家], written by Ba Jin [巴金] and published in 1933 (McDougall and Louie 1997). Contemporary mainland Chinese films, such as Zhang Yuan's *Sons* mentioned in Chapter 4 (Knight 2006), carry on this tradition, as do contemporary mainland Chinese television serial dramas (Kong 2008; Xu 2008). According to Zhu *et al.* (2008), contemporary television serial dramas about 'everyday life' (9) in mainland

China represent 'a powerful story-telling medium' (3), whose popularity to the mainland Chinese audience now rivals that of film. A factor in this success, Zhu *et al.* (2008, 3) point out, is that 'Chinese television drama draws many of its codes, conventions, and narrative strategies from cinema.' As such, the stories told in these dramas, like the stories told in film, commonly engage the salient 'cultural debates' occurring in contemporary mainland Chinese society (Zhu *et al.* 2008, 13). Caring for parents in their old age, especially in illness, comprises one of the 'ethical dilemmas and moral conflicts' (Kong 2008, 83) commonly faced by the contemporary urban family in an ageing society such as mainland China (see Chapters 1 and 5). This is particularly the case given the increasing nuclearity of the urban family, due, in part, to the one-child policy, and the increasing demands that socioeconomic reform has placed on those who traditionally are expected to care for the elderly (Cook and Dong 2011).

Chinese cultural norms traditionally assign caregiving-for-the-elderly duties to women family members (Ikels 1998; Zhan 2006). Both productions under study recount stories of women caring for elderly family members with dementia, one a daughter and the other a daughter-in-law. The experiences of women caring for elderly family members with dementia draw attention to the challenges of family life and family relations in contemporary urban mainland China, in that mainland Chinese women are still expected to manage the competing demands of a career and a family (Cook and Dong 2011; Croll 1995; Guo 2010; Kong 2008; Korabik 1993; Mann 2011). This is despite the advances in the position of women brought about by the communist government since 1949 (Cook and Dong 2011; Croll 1995; Korabik 1993; Roberts 2010).

As in Chapter 4, the ensuing analysis focuses not on the social and political critique contained in the film and television serial drama under study but on how the stories of the two women characters caring for elderly family members with dementia are culturally shaped. The individual stories of the two women are separated out from the broader plots of each of the productions and then examined in terms of the meanings that emerge through the temporal and causal ordering of life events, through the claiming and refashioning of identities, and through language use. The analysis distinguishes commonalities in and differences between how culture shapes the life stories of family caregiving in dementia analysed in Chapter 5 and how culture shapes the filmic stories analysed in the current chapter. The ensuing analysis also identifies the prevailing meta-narrative of family caregiving in dementia circulating in Chinese communities, which is drawn on in the productions under study.

Analysis of *Gone is the One Who Held Me Dearest in the World*

Gone is the One Who Held Me Dearest in the World is a 2002 film by mainland Chinese woman director, Ma Xiaoying [马晓颖]. This was her debut production as a film director (Vanderstaay 2011). The film is of the 'sixth generation' type (see Chapter 4) and comprises one of a number of recent films by female directors in mainland China which explore the 'mother-daughter relationship'

(Vanderstaay 2011, 69). The film is based on the 1994 autobiographical novel of the same name written by renowned mainland Chinese female literary author, Zhang Jie [张洁].[1] Both film and novel explore the 'frequently contentious relationship' (Vanderstaay 2011, 68) between a daughter, a successful literary writer who is suddenly thrown into a caregiving role, and her mother, who for the first time in her life finds herself highly dependent on her daughter's care when she is diagnosed with advanced dementia-related brain atrophy and a comorbid brain tumour. The issue of dementia, while important in the film, remains subordinate throughout the film to the primary critique of family life and family relations in contemporary urban mainland China, in particular the relations between a confident, successful, 'new urban' Chinese woman and her elderly mother.

The daughter's story

The story begins with a flash-forward to the mother's death, centring on the daughter's profound grief. The daughter blames herself for what she sees as the untimely and undeserved passing of her mother: 'Mother died a wrongful death' [妈是含冤而死的]. She laments, 'it was I who harmed Mother; it was my obstinacy that caused the death of Mother; it was I who strangled Mother.' [是我害了妈, 是我的刚愎自用害死了妈, 是我把妈勒死的]. She sees herself as having failed in the caregiving role, having been powerless, in the end, to control the course of her mother's illness: 'I failed … I could not prevail over fate and could not prevail over God.' [我失败了 … 我不可战胜命运, 也不可战胜上帝]. Her failure and helplessness in being unable to ward off her mother's terminal decline in the face of dementia are contrasted with images of her professional success, travelling the globe and being mobbed by fans at a book signing event. These images of professional diligence and accomplishment, in turn, are contrasted with images of her home life, draped in an apron busy with housework and dutifully caring for her husband on his return from work. Her conflicted performance of the normative role for women in Chinese culture becomes clear as the daughter proceeds to visit her elderly mother, who lives separately in a traditional alleyway (*hutong*) [胡同] precinct. The mother is cared for by paid help, a young girl from the countryside, likely a relative, who seems more aware of the mother's day-to-day concerns and issues than the daughter. Despite having a fulltime nanny [保姆], the mother looks dishevelled and unkempt in appearance. The nanny informs the daughter that 'These days Granny has been getting confused all the time' [姥姥最近老发糊涂] as well as talking to herself and seeing things. The daughter is surprised by this revelation and the revelation that her mother has lost her formerly voracious appetite [现在呀, 眼小肚子也小了]. There is an inference that the daughter should have noticed these changes herself, if she had been paying proper attention to her mother. This subsequently materialises in expressions of guilt by the daughter: 'I can be considered to be deeply unfilial. When she was most in need of me to be by her side I abandoned her from afar.' [我算是大不孝了. 在她最需要我左右一旁的时候我却远远的把她丢下了].

On the advice of a friend, the daughter takes her mother to a hospital for tests for what she believes is primarily an issue with her mother's vision. We then find the daughter working in her mother's home, where she soon encounters some of her mother's less desirable habits, such as hoarding fruit and using an old rag rather than toilet paper when toileting herself. The daughter's reaction is far from considered. She severely scolds her mother for these behaviours: 'No wonder my father did not care about you. I don't think anyone who's living with you could put up with it.' [怪不得我爸不愿理您，我看谁跟您在一起都受不了]. Soon the daughter obtains the results of her mother's medical tests: the mother has progressive 'brain atrophy' [脑萎缩] and a comorbid brain tumour. While the tumour is operable, the doctor concedes that there is absolutely nothing he can do about the dementia [脑萎缩就毫无办法了], which, he warns, will inevitably leave her in a vegetative state [和植物人一样]. Receiving no support from her husband, and with her own daughter studying in the United States, the daughter follows medical advice to admit her mother to the hospital. While in the past, she recalls, her mother, when ill, had dealt with everything by herself [就是有病，常常是独自面对一切], this time it was her responsibility to arrange and finance the hospitalisation.

Having hospitalised her mother, the daughter has a conference with the treating surgeon who warns of the operative risks for someone of her mother's age. The doctor implores the daughter to make the decision over whether or not to proceed with the tumour surgery, but, to his dismay, the daughter insists on leaving the decision to her mother. The professional expectation, in Chinese culture, is that the family members would make medical decisions on behalf of elderly parents. As it turns out, the mother is adamant that she wants to undergo surgery for the tumour, as not doing so could result in blindness, a state she is not willing to entertain [我不愿意那样活着].

Images of the daughter undertaking caregiving and home duties come to dominate her story: planning her daughter's wedding gown for the following year's wedding, bathing her mother in the hospital, shopping, washing the family car, collecting her in-laws from the railway station, choosing a head scarf to cover her mother's preoperatively shaved head and sleeping overnight in the hospital with her mother. Postoperatively, the daughter remains in the hospital, working from her laptop and caring for her recuperating mother. The surgery is a success but, unfortunately, the signs of dementia progressively worsen with the mother experiencing delusions, confusion and urinary urgency. The daughter remains unsure whether the mother is deliberately behaving in a difficult manner or whether it is a manifestation of her illness. She begins to openly question her mother: 'You are no longer sick, so why do you still torment people?' [您都没病了，您怎么还折腾人啊?]. It is to no avail as the mother's behaviour becomes increasingly demanding. Tested more and more, the daughter, nevertheless, does not indulge the mother, with frequent conflict arising between the pair. The essence of their relationship is brought into scrutiny: 'In short, at that time it seemed as if Mother and I had been cursed. I was not a daughter who dearly loved her mother and Mother was not a mother who dearly loved me.' [总之，那

时我和妈就像中了邪. 我不是挚爱妈的女儿, 妈也不是挚爱我的妈妈]. The mother's dementia, nevertheless, is still seen by the daughter to underpin the difficult behaviours: 'In fact, how was Mother a tormentor; her illness had brought on self-torment.' [其实, 妈哪是折腾人, 她是病得开始折腾自己了].

When the mother's behaviour becomes too disruptive for the hospital staff, the daughter has little choice but to take her mother back to her home to care for her. The daughter expresses some frustration at this outcome. Yet, interspersed with the frosty images of the daughter's exhaustion and dissatisfaction are the tender images of the pair at home, grooming each other's hair and sharing a bottle of fine wine. At first, being cared for in the luxury of the daughter's home, in stark contrast to the sterility of the hospital ward, projects an element of warmth and security about the mother's circumstances, despite the gravity of her, thus far, not openly spoken about dementia. Over time, however, the mother's gradual functional decline and attendant reluctance to engage in activities and self-care come to concern the daughter. The doctor advises the daughter to force the mother to be active, lest her idleness hasten her dementia-induced decline [你越是不让她做, 就越是害了她]. The daughter responds by forcing the mother to be active and take care of her own personal needs such as toileting, without assistance from the nanny or herself. Only this way can the mother's dementia, now openly spoken about by the daughter, be warded off.

The daughter's methods to encourage activity by the mother border on abuse. The daughter threatens leaving the door to the bathroom open when the husband is at home in order to motivate the mother to promptly toilet herself. She rather callously shows her mother the radiographic scans demonstrating the severity of the brain atrophy brought on by her dementia and warns her mother that continuing her present behaviour will greatly hasten her death [照这样下去, 不过三个月你就死了]. She brusquely hurries her mother along a walking path in the local park despite the mother's obvious distress, claiming that the mother walks too slowly. As such, the daughter sees herself as fully implementing the doctor's advice, to the benefit of the mother.

Yet, despite this apparent commitment to the care of her mother, the daughter voluntarily takes a week to travel to Sweden to take part in a literary awards ceremony, leaving her mother in the care of a local kindergarten that doubles as an aged care centre. In the aged care centre the mother is sullen. Left alone in her wheelchair, we see her through the wire fence surrounding the compound, staring listlessly at a tree or peering aimlessly through the main gate. On her return, traces of guilt begin to re-enter the daughter's thoughts: 'I give thought to others all day long, but rarely give thought to my own mother.' [我终日为别人着想, 却很少为自己妈着想]. It is clear from this outcome that her mother's care should be wholly undertaken in the home setting and not be consigned to institutions.

Back in the daughter's home after her return from Sweden, the mother has noticeably deteriorated. Despite protestations by her mother, the daughter proceeds to deny the mother's condition: 'Mother, following your [tumour] surgery you're not ill anymore. All is well with the world.' [妈呀, 您做完手术以

后啊都没病了 … 一切万事大吉]. The daughter looks to medicine to justify her stance: 'I trust science; I trust the doctors.' [我信科学，我信大夫们]. Accordingly, she places blame for the mother's loss of mobility on her failure to keep active and not the illness: 'Mother, this way, is giving up on herself. It's simply a betrayal of my love and a betrayal of our common suffering and hardship.' [妈这样做是自暴自弃，简直是对我爱的背叛，是对我们共同的苦难艰辛的背叛].

Gradually, however, the daughter begins to question the effectiveness of her approach to caregiving: 'All the efforts she and I have made, could it be that they've all come to nothing? Could it be that they are all not capable of saving Mother?' [我和她所做的一切努力，难道都是一场空？难道都救不了她吗？]. With the mother's condition continuing to deteriorate she can now only feebly crawl on the floor to go to the bathroom. The daughter insists she stand and walk, but her mother's attempts only exhaust her and she momentarily blacks out. From this moment on the daughter abandons her efforts to keep her mother active. We now find the pair at peace with each other, quietly enjoying each other's company on the sofa where the mother sleeps. With this, the mother soon passes away.

Discussion

Similar to the life stories analysed in Chapter 5, dementia marks a temporal juncture in the family caregiver's (and her mother's) life. Unlike the life stories analysed in Chapter 5, however, this juncture *does* equate to a turbulent 'biographical disruption' for the family caregiver (Bury 1982, 169). As a consequence, the larger narrative focus in the filmic story under study, which is diverted to the ill family member in the life story counterparts, returns to recount the challenges and upheaval faced by the family caregiver.

The tumult experienced by the daughter stems from her public identity as a modern, highly successful Chinese career woman, whose creative writing talent is nationally and internationally acclaimed. She is independent and unencumbered in her day-to-day life. Her only child is studying in the United States. Her only living parent lives separately, cared for by a live-in nanny which she pays for. She visits the mother whenever she can amidst a busy schedule. She is fully engaged and enmeshed in her professional endeavours. Dementia, however, arrives to disrupt this and obliges her to meet the cultural expectation to care for the ill mother in her home.

The daughter is not wholly unequipped to meet this 'moral challenge' (see Chapter 5). She displays some traces of normative womanhood in Chinese culture by undertaking household chores, making preparations for her own daughter's wedding, and dutifully taking care of her husband's every need in the home (Guo 2010; Roberts 2010). What is more, at times she defers to men, for example, by dutifully picking up her in-laws from the railway station downtown on her husband's insistence, even though her own mother is undergoing surgery on this day. Also on her husband's insistence, she places her mother in institutional care when she travels overseas. She also willingly complies with the male doctor's advice that her mother needs to undergo what constitutes life-endangering surgery. Thus, amidst her presentation as a modern Chinese woman, culturally normative elements remain on display, with men in her world emerging as peripheral power figures who remain external to her drama yet continue to impact on it.

This liminal identity performed by the daughter, which asserts modern Chinese womanhood, characterised by productivity and independence, yet concurrently accedes to normative roles for women in Chinese culture, is emblematic of the position of mainland Chinese women in the post-Mao reform period (Cook and Dong 2011; Guo 2010; Kong 2008; Korabik 1993; Mann 2011). Croll (1995, 9) states that, despite the great advances in women's educational and professional status during this period, 'many Chinese women have found themselves still strongly bound by inherited rhetorical shackles and by their straddling of old and new.' Korabik (1993, 49) argues that this demonstrates that the mainland Chinese government's 'attempt to achieve equality through the economic emancipation of women has met with only limited success …. [T]he Chinese Communist Party has neither successfully eliminated the remnants of feudal thinking, nor implemented a viable feminist theory.' The one-child policy and ready access to child care may have facilitated women's entry into the workforce in mainland China, yet, Korabik (1993, 60, 62) states, 'a patriarchal division of labor in which household tasks … [including] elder care … are relegated to women still exists, with women's domestic roles viewed as equal to or more important than their careers.' Guo's (2010) analysis of a 2006 campaign undertaken by the All-China Women's Federation and other party-state affiliated agencies confirms this, with the campaign characterising 'exemplary mothers' (52) as 'independent and self-supporting career women' who displayed 'industriousness and frugality in running the household' (49) and 'a strong sense of duty to the family' (50), alongside other qualities such as patriotism, support for the communist party and 'a strong sense of social responsibility' (49).

In the filmic story under study, the unsustainability of this liminal identity is exposed when the modern Chinese woman is shouldered with the burden of caring for an elderly parent with dementia. The daughter looks to normative womanhood of 'old' (Croll 1995, 9) to perform her family caregiving role, traces of which she continues to act out in her day-to-day life in the home setting. Yet, in the daughter's story, her normative womanhood, diluted by her ardent sense of modernity, is found to be inadequate for successfully carrying out the family caregiving role. She experiences no compensatory feelings of poise and serenity. What is more, the family caregiving role falls to her alone. Men assign her this role, as is culturally normative (Ikels 1998; Zhan 2006), but provide little support in its execution (Guo 2010). As a consequence, the daughter is left to face the frustration and anger when a facet of the modernity that she so values and which so strongly informs her sense of self, namely, biomedicine, is unable to ward off the mother's dementia-related decline and, so, ease the burden of family caregiving.

In the filmic story under study, the unsustainability of the daughter's liminal identity in family caregiving in dementia is contrasted with the effectiveness of the nanny's sense of self. In the story, the nanny comes to serve as a reference point alongside which the daughter is measured, primarily, as wanting. The nanny is a rural girl who fully displays the qualities of normative womanhood in Chinese culture. She is modest in attire and unassuming and composed in temperament. The daughter, in contrast, wears stylish attire and is assertive and, at times, unconventional and stubborn in temperament. She is often angry with her ill mother and insists, for example, on including her mother in the decision over whether to operate on the comorbid tumour, in contravention of cultural norms. The nanny works in a feminised, humble vocation. The daughter, on the other hand, is a career professional, whose occupation outclasses her husband's. The nanny, supposedly in an ancillary caregiving role, devotes all her efforts to making the mother as comfortable as possible as she progressively deteriorates. The daughter, having assumed the primary caregiving role, in contrast, is often seen working on her laptop in the mother's room. She also elects to institutionalise the mother, albeit on her husband's insistence, when she chooses to go on an overseas trip despite the state of the mother's health.

The foremost distinction between the daughter and the nanny lies in the explanatory models that they embrace in the face of the mother's decline. The nanny treats the mother's condition as normative decline in old age, in line with the cultural explanation identified in Chapter 5. The daughter, however, biomedicalises the mother's condition. Two opposing explanatory models of dementia, therefore, contend in the daughter's story: dementia as pathology amenable to structured intervention (biomedical) versus dementia as normative old age (cultural). The sophisticated urban professional, who personifies modern notions of Chinese womanhood, embraces the former and the language that characterises it ('brain atrophy' [脑萎缩]). The simple nanny from the countryside, who personifies more traditional notions of Chinese womanhood, embraces the latter and the language of everyday life (Mishler 1984). The biomedical model, however, merely causes the daughter great stress and frustration as her exhortations and interventions, as counselled by the health professionals, bring about little obvious improvement in the mother and only serve to cause the mother further discomfort. At first, the daughter accuses the mother of 'not responding well' when her exhortations and interventions fail to ward off the mother's decline, echoing the cultural stigma attached to 'not ageing well' (see Chapter 5). This quickly turns to self-blame, in contrast to the nanny who, like the family caregivers in dementia whose life stories were analysed in Chapter 5, can readily locate blame in 'age itself' (Hinton *et al.* 2000, 126). Biomedicine, thus, fails the daughter and only adds to her sense of burden and culpability. The nanny, in contrast, enjoys a smooth and fond relationship with the mother as she dotingly caters to the mother's every whim and urge, just like a child. This is just as cultural norms would prescribe (see Chapter 5).

The daughter's biomedicalisation of dementia befits the urbane and intellectual sophistication of her identity as a modern Chinese woman. It also compels her to look to the future to sustain her family caregiving endeavour. Biomedicine promises (partial) remedy and remedy is future oriented (Frank 1995). For the daughter, the past signifies regret and self-blame for the professed neglect of her ageing mother in bygone years. In contrast to the life stories of family caregiving in dementia, therefore, memories of the embodied person from before the onset of illness are not revived in the filmic story under study. The future (remedy) rather than the past (memory) is drawn on to sustain the family caregiving endeavour. This, as noted above, only leads to frustration, anger, heartache and self-blame when biomedicine's promise of remedy is not met. In the filmic story under study, poise and serenity are only found when biomedicine's promise, and along with it the daughter's modernity, are relinquished and the company of the mother is innocently enjoyed as she approaches the end of her life journey.

In sum, biomedicalisation of dementia in the filmic story under study leads to the family caregiver looking to the future (remedy) rather than the past (memory) to sustain her family caregiving endeavour. This befits her identity as a modern Chinese woman, a liminal construct that 'straddl[es]' the 'old and new' (Croll 1995, 9). This identity is problematic in meeting the moral challenge presented by family caregiving in dementia. The 'new' (modernity) exacerbates the biographical disruption that family caregiving in dementia presents and fails to ward off illness-related decline. The traces of 'old' (normative womanhood in Chinese culture) are insufficient to provide compensatory feelings of poise and composure. Only by fuller embracing of the 'old', as personified by the nanny, can the daughter temper the disruption and tumult that she experiences in meeting the moral challenge of family caregiving in dementia.

Analysis of *Watch for the Happiness*

Watch for the Happiness is a 2005 22-part television serial drama by prolific mainland Chinese television series director Zeng Xiaoxin [曾晓欣]. The production is based on the 2005 novel Feng Ji [疯祭] by lesser known mainland Chinese author Zhai Enmeng [翟恩猛]. Both director and author are men. The television drama recounts a family's struggle to manage the care for their recently widowed elderly mother who begins to display signs of dementia. The mother has three children, two living in the city and one in the countryside. Her care for the most part falls to the younger, highly educated, well-off son and his wife living in the city, both professionals. The mother had already been living with the young couple for a number of years. The other two children, who step in temporarily to provide care, are quite poor and less educated, one running a small local store and the other a farmer. The issue of dementia, while important in the television drama, primarily constitutes a means by which to critique, in greater depth, family life and family relations in contemporary mainland China, in particular the relations between siblings and a husband and wife caring for an elderly mother with dementia.

The daughter-in-law's story

The television drama begins, as it ends, with generations of the family coming together, initially, to celebrate the family patriarch's eightieth birthday. The patriarch falls ill before arriving at the event and subsequently dies. The production cuts to a month later to the home of the younger son, Tianshu [天书], and his wife, Xiangyu [香雨], with whom the parents had been residing for a number of years. Tianshu is a successful university professor and Xiangyu a middle school teacher. Their comfortable financial status is evident in their large city apartment. In the apartment, the mother remains visibly traumatised by her husband's recent death, as Tianshu's siblings discuss her future living arrangements. Amidst these discussions the question of a large amount of life savings held by the mother and father arises. The mother accuses Xiangyu, who has dutifully fulfilled the normative role of a daughter-in-law in Chinese culture (Ikels 1998; Zhan 2006), being the primary caregiver for the parents over the past years, of having taken their life savings. As Tianshu's siblings quarrel over the disappearance of the savings, the mother mysteriously vanishes. Tianshu and his siblings believe that the mother has left due to mistreatment of her by Xiangyu. Amidst these accusations, Xiangyu is determined to find the mother. After a lengthy search, the mother is eventually located aimlessly wandering in a nearby village. She had been looking for a daughter, now deceased, who she had given up as a child during a time of famine long ago.

Recovering in hospital, the mother is diagnosed with dementia, a condition for which the treating psychiatrist ominously warns 'there is unlikely to be any particularly good treatment. This kind of illness, well, is a form of torment for the ill person and the family …. Nursing an elderly person with dementia will bring any kind of family into total chaos.' [我想也不会有什么特别好的治疗办法, 这种病啊对病人本身和家人都是一种折磨 … 护理一个患痴呆病的老人什么样的家庭都会被搞得乱了套]. The psychiatrist advises the family to place the mother in an aged care home, yet, without any discussion with his wife, Tianshu rejects the idea outright: 'We will not send her to an aged care home; this is simply not possible. With my, my mother in this situation, we cannot allow her to leave our home, let alone send her to an aged care home.' [不是送敬老院, 这根本不可能. 我, 我母亲这种情况, 我们是不可能让她离开家的, 更不会把她送到敬老院]. He draws on his mother's past suffering to justify this duty to continue to care for her in the home: '[Mother], having endured difficulty until all her children had married and started a career, precisely, ought to enjoy a peaceful and comfortable life.' [好不容易熬到儿女们都成家立业了, 这正是应该享点儿清福].

While Tianshu is resolute in his decision to care for his mother in the home, day-to-day care falls to Xiangyu, as was the case before the mother had fallen ill. The mother soon becomes publicly disruptive, for example, collecting leaves from the upper branches of trees in the public garden at the front of the apartment complex where they live, believing that there is no food left to eat at home [咱撸点儿树叶子家里没吃的啦]. Amidst the shame that the public display of bizarre behaviour brings (see Chapter 3), Tianshu proceeds to blame Xiangyu for allowing the mother to slip away from her sight while caring for her at home. Although hurt, and despite the difficulties already faced in trying to care for the mother at home, Xiangyu rejects her urbane and wealthy younger sister's advice to place the mother in an aged care facility. Xiangyu feels beholden to the mother:

> My mother-in-law is most fond of me. Before I couldn't even cook; she shouldered large and small matters in the home on her own. In my heart I truly could not bear to, as you say, send her to an aged care home. [我婆婆最 疼我, 以前我连饭都不会做, 家里大大小小的事都是她一个人担着. 你要说 把她送到养老院, 我真是于心不忍].

As time goes by Xiangyu becomes increasingly stressed by the burden of caring for the mother as well as continuing with her regular household duties and her middle school teaching. Nevertheless, she does not seek respite from this burden, for example, by asking her husband to also take some time off from work to care for his mother. The husband merely suggests locking the mother inside the apartment when Xiangyu has to go to work during the daytime. Against her instincts, Xiangyu follows this advice and, in addition, follows the psychiatrist's advice by sedating the mother when she leaves home. Unfortunately, she marginally overdoses the mother and, on her return, is unable to rouse the mother from her sleep, causing her much distress. Tianshu consoles his wife, observing that being filial is a challenge: 'This filial piety, ah, it's, well, easier said than done.' [这个孝啊, 是说起来容易做起来难哪]. He continues to counsel locking his mother in the home when he and his wife must be absent, until the mother is found one day by Tianshu's brother in great distress as a result of being locked up alone in the home. This results in Tianshu's actions being strongly criticised by his siblings.

Recognising that the mother cannot be left unaccompanied in the home, Tianshu begins to provide some respite for Xiangyu by spending more time at home with the mother during the day. Fearing, however, that the mother is being mistreated by Tianshu and Xiangyu, Tianshu's sister moves the mother to her home, believing that she can provide better care. The sister's attentive care is seen to bring a marked improvement in the mother's condition, such that she refutes Tianshu and Xiangyu's biomedicalisation of the mother's deemed unusual behaviour as dementia:

> You said that Mother was like this and that. How is it that I did not notice any of this? Look, Mother is fine … You cannot trust a doctor's remarks. Even when there's no illness he can still speak of some illness. [你说妈又这 了又那了. 我咋一点儿都没看出来呀. 你看妈好好的 … 大夫那话你就不能 信, 没病他也能给你说出点儿病来呀].

Soon after, however, the mother's symptoms return and Tianshu's sister acknowledges the burden that Tianshu and Xiangyu had faced in caring for the mother: 'This illness our mother has, well, places a lot of burden on a person. I'd rather look after ten children than look after a mad mother.' [咱妈这病多拖累人哪, 宁看十个孩子不看一个疯妈]. The sister relinquishes care of the mother to Tianshu and Xiangyu when she herself becomes seriously ill with diabetes.

This time, Tianshu and Xiangyu employ a nanny [保姆] to help them care for the mother at home, but the nanny does not last. She is unwilling to care for a 'mad-person': 'I can keep an old person company … but not a madwoman.' [我是会陪老人说话 … 陪个疯子说话, 我可不会]. A second nanny, similarly, does not last. A third nanny, employed by Xiangyu, is secretly abusive to the mother. Xiangyu eventually walks in on the nanny abusing the mother and throws her out. Xiangyu is left to take the blame from her husband's siblings for allowing the nanny to abuse the mother. Moreover, to make matters worse, the mother, deluded, subsequently believes that Xiangyu is the nanny and becomes violently agitated when Xiangyu tries to care for her. The situation further worsens when the mother comes to view Xiangyu as a 'bandit' [胡子]. Xiangyu is no longer able to be anywhere near the mother, let alone adequately provide care for her in the home. She must surreptitiously move around her own home, continuing to undertake household duties, yet avoiding contact with the mother. In the end, due to Xiangyu's negative effect on an increasingly deluded mother, as well as her own daughter's plummeting grades at school, Xiangyu decides, on her own accord, to move out of home with her daughter: 'For Mother's sake, for our child's sake, and for our own sake, tomorrow I'll start looking for an apartment to go to.' [明天我就去找房子去, 为了妈、为了孩子、也为了我们自己]. She leaves Tianshu to manage caring for his mother on his own.

Xiangyu moves into a run-down courtyard dwelling in a poor alleyway (*hutong*) [胡同] precinct near her daughter's school. She believes this choice of residence will allow her and Tianshu to save some money for their daughter's future university education as well as for any contingencies that may await them as the mother's condition progressively deteriorates. Living apart, however, damages Xiangyu's relationship with her husband and she begins to suspect him of having an intimate relationship with the mother's psychiatrist. The psychiatrist had taken a keen interest in the care of the mother, regularly visiting her at home. One day, Xiangyu returns to the family apartment and confronts her husband about his relationship with the psychiatrist. The mother, as before, is terrified by Xiangyu's presence, still believing that she is a bandit. Xiangyu, however, refuses to leave the apartment, despite the mother's obvious distress. Tianshu pleads for Xiangyu to leave the home in order to allow the mother to settle down, however, Xiangyu resolutely stands her ground. In desperation Tianshu slaps Xiangyu to force her to leave.

Despite being beaten by Tianshu and refusing to speak with him when he seeks her out, Xiangyu continues to dutifully bring food to the apartment for the mother. Recognising the chaos afflicting Tianshu's household, his siblings organise for the mother to go and live in the countryside with her older son. With the mother having left the home, and following the psychiatrist's assurance that she and Tianshu are not having a relationship, Xiangyu returns home to the family apartment, repentant for the earlier incident in front of the mother and for mistakenly believing that her husband was having an affair with the psychiatrist: 'I am also to blame in this matter; without clarifying things I just blindly argued.' [这事也怪我，没搞清楚就瞎嚷嚷]. She willingly goes back to her regular household duties.

On hearing that the mother is now causing disorder in Tianshu's older brother's home, Xiangyu suggests sending the mother to an aged care home. Tianshu continues to refuse to do this. However, when the older brother dies suddenly, the mother is reluctantly placed in a dementia-care hospice. Tianshu's sister has now formed the same view as Xiangyu: 'We cannot on account of Mother throw our own lives away.' [我们不能因为妈把我们自己的生活都给抛掉吧]. The mother's condition rapidly deteriorates in the hospice, such that she does not recognise family members anymore and becomes incontinent. The hospice staff insist that this merely reflects the normative deterioration experienced in dementia. When the mother has a fall when unattended in the toilet, however, Tianshu takes her back home, telling Xiangyu that he will resign from his current position in the university and take care of the mother fulltime himself. Xiangyu accedes to her husband's decision, however, she is eventually drawn back into caring for the mother when the mother refuses to allow Tianshu to change her diaper and bathe her.

The decision to bring the mother back home is seemingly validated by a dramatic improvement in her condition, counter to the continuing decline foreshadowed by the psychiatrist in hospital. Encouraged by this, Tianshu espouses the virtues of being filial, telling his nephew 'Granma is old and muddled now. Can we turn our back on her? Previously Granma took care of us, now we take care of her. This is only the right and proper thing to do.' [现在姥姥老了、糊涂了，嫌弃她了是不是啊. 过去是姥姥照顾我们，现在是我们照顾姥姥，这都是天经地义的事情]. However, such talk only serves to make Xiangyu feel guilty about having dinner out with her sister while her husband remains at home tending to his mother. While in the public garden with Tianshu and Xiangyu's daughter, the mother disappears and Xiangyu is angered when Tianshu admonishes his daughter for being inattentive. Although the mother is eventually found, the chastised daughter had run away and is almost kidnapped by criminals trafficking in women, leaving her psychologically traumatised by the experience.

For the second time, Xiangyu decides to move out of the family apartment so as to protect her child. In the end, however, Xiangyu returns home with her daughter after her younger sister reminds her of the value of having a responsible husband like Tianshu [有责任心的男人才是好男人]. With Xiangyu and her daughter back at home with Tianshu and his mother, the extended family reunites to celebrate the occasion. The mother, however, has a bad fall. Later in hospital the psychiatrist informs the family that the mother's condition is now end-stage. A surprisingly lucid mother expresses her deep indebtedness to Xiangyu for the care she has given her over the years: 'Everyone has their strong points. Living with you these years, I have had a happy and prosperous life. My youngest son taking you as his wife is, well, his good fortune and my good fortune.' [十个手指

头还不一边儿长呢, 妈这些年跟着你过, 妈享福了, 我老疙瘩娶了你这个媳妇啊, 是他的福分儿, 也是妈的福气]. The mother then requests to be taken back to her birth village to die. Here, the television drama concludes, with the generations of the family accompanying the mother home to her final resting place.

Discussion

Dementia marks a temporal juncture in the family caregiver's life in the filmic story under study. It does not, however, equate to the tumultuous 'biographical disruption' experienced by the daughter in *Gone is the One Who Held Me Dearest in the World* (Bury 1982, 169). The daughter-in-law, like the daughter, is presented as a modern Chinese woman, holding down a career as a middle school teacher in addition to managing the day-to-day running of her household. The daughter-in-law, however, has already been taking care of her elderly in-laws in the home for a number of years, so caring for a suddenly ill mother-in-law, despite the unique challenges this presents, ostensibly represents a continuation of her life circumstance.

The daughter-in-law approaches caring for the mother when she falls ill in a way that allows her, in the end, to attain a more moral and reconciled position than the daughter in *Gone is the One Who Held Me Dearest in the World*. One reason for this is, from the outset of her story, Xiangyu is presented as more culturally equipped to meet the 'moral challenge' of caring for the ill mother in the home setting. While also a modern Chinese woman holding down a career, she is much more consistent and seamless in her performance of normative womanhood in Chinese culture. As mentioned, she has successfully cared for her elderly in-laws in the home for a number of years. As such, her record of filiality is unblemished (Guo 2010). Xiangyu is also diligently raising her teenage daughter at home. In *Gone is the One Who Held Me Dearest in the World*, her counterpart's daughter has been sent overseas to study, leaving few opportunities in the counterpart's story to view her in her role as a mother (Guo 2010). In addition, Xiangyu works in a highly feminised, 'respectable' profession (Guo 2010, 59) that provides a modest income in mainland China, while, in accordance with cultural norms, her husband works in a profession of higher social status and with higher remuneration. The daughter in *Gone is the One Who Held Me Dearest in the World*, on the other hand, works in a 'glamorous' but not a traditionally feminine profession (Guo 2010, 59), with an income that likely exceeds that of her husband.

Xiangyu's identity in the filmic story under study does not vacillate in the interstices between modernity and normative womanhood in Chinese culture, as does her counterpart's in *Gone is the One Who Held Me Dearest in the World*. While her counterpart was unable to comfortably reconcile her two subjective positionings 'straddling' the 'old and new' (Croll 1995, 9), Xiangyu prioritises the former (Korabik 1993). She does so while maintaining her modern credentials in a way that the nanny in her counterpart's story, who personifies normative Chinese womanhood, does not. Xiangyu is an educated professional.

She does not frame the mother's decline as normative ageing, as her husband's siblings do, but unhesitatingly biomedicalises it as dementia. She holds to her modern beliefs and the health professional's advice, even though they lead her husband's siblings to openly question her moral standing for quite a period of time. They believe that the mother is just old, not 'mad'. Xiangyu, nevertheless, is able to maintain her moral standing for the duration of the story under study, unlike her counterpart in *Gone is the One Who Held Me Dearest in the World*, through her more consistent and seamless performance of normative Chinese womanhood. She adeptly carries out her duties as a daughter-in-law, tending to the needs of her co-resident in-laws and, later, her ill mother-in-law; her normative duties as a wife, cooking, cleaning and providing for her husband; and her normative duties as a mother, nurturing and protecting her teenage daughter. For the most part, she carries out these duties without questioning and in deference to her husband, even when her husband and his siblings wrongfully point out what they believe to be failings in the ways she has carried them out.

Where Xiangyu seemingly breaks from the cultural script, for example, in twice abandoning the care of the ill mother to her husband, it is only because there is a greater moral priority in play, namely, protection of her child. Such breaches do not result from her seeking to further her career or for personal gain, as is the case in *Gone is the One Who Held Me Dearest in the World*. Xiangyu also preserves her moral standing on these occasions by her self-sacrifice in choosing to live in humble conditions in order to save money for any future contingencies for her daughter and the ill mother; by continuing to bring food to the family home for the ill mother, even after a beating from her husband; by eventually returning to the family home on each occasion after a short period of time; and by expressing regret for her transgressions on her return and willingly returning to family caregiving duties for the ill mother. Thus, in Xiangyu's story, any apparent moral transgression quickly meets with exoneration (Bury 2001).

Xiangyu's steady and largely culturally coherent performance of family caregiving in dementia is contrasted with the inconsistent and self-contradictory performances of her poor and uneducated sister-in-law and her urbane and wealthy younger sister. Her sister-in-law, who runs a small corner stall, at the outset more fully personifies the normative response in Chinese culture, in denying that the mother has a biomedical condition (see Chapter 5). Moreover, on taking on care of the mother in her own home, the sister-in-law is even willing to allow her young grandson, who lives in the home together with his divorced father, to be taken away and placed with the grandson's estranged mother, in accordance with a court order that cites the risk presented to the grandson in sharing the home with his unruly, demented great-grandmother. Yet, the sister-in-law's deeply filial behaviour transforms to apparent culturally-informed disdain (the 'mad mother' [疯妈]),[2] when she finally resigns herself to the biomedical origin of her mother's condition and accepts the need for her to be institutionalised. On the other hand, Xiangyu's younger sister, who runs a very successful exclusive boutique downtown, at the outset more fully personifies the 'modern' response in advocating institutionalisation of the ill mother. Yet, by the end of the story, she is advising Xiangyu to return home with her daughter to live with Tianshu and the ill mother, as she now views Tianshu as 'responsible' [有责任心] in light of his devotion to the ill mother and his wife. This is despite the fact that he had previously beaten Xiangyu. Throughout the filmic story under study, therefore, Xiangyu steadily occupies the moral ground in her performance of family caregiving in dementia, being situated subjectively between her sister-in-law and her younger sister and their, ultimately self-contradictory, personifications of 'old and new' (Croll 1995, 9).

In biomedicalising the mother's decline as dementia, Xiangyu does not engage biomedicine's promise of remedy to sustain her in the family caregiving endeavour, as does the daughter in *Gone is the One Who Held Me Dearest in the World*. Xiangyu, instead, turns to positive memories of the mother before illness to sustain her in caregiving, as did the family caregivers in the life stories analysed in Chapter 5. The key difference between Xiangyu and her counterpart in *Gone is the One Who Held Me Dearest in the World* lies in Xiangyu's capacity to draw on such memories without concurrently triggering any sense of self-blame over failing to be filial to the mother in years gone by. As a result, Xiangyu largely avoids the extreme frustration, anger and heartache that her counterpart experiences in *Gone is the One Who Held Me Dearest in the World* in looking to the future (remedy) to sustain her family caregiving endeavour.

All in all, biomedicine plays an ambivalent role in the filmic story under study. Xiangyu's biomedicalisation of the mother's decline as dementia is a sign of her modernity. This constitutes a positive trait in the story, when compared to her husband's less educated siblings. Yet, Xiangyu does not draw on biomedicine's promise of remedy, as her counterpart does in *Gone is the One Who Held Me Dearest in the World*, to sustain her in family caregiving in dementia. She seemingly follows culturally normative practice in reviving positive memories of the embodied person from before. What is more, biomedicine does not assuage the problems faced by Xiangyu in caring for the ill mother, but only exacerbates them. Medication prescribed by the psychiatrist dangerously over-sedates the mother. The mother's condition rapidly deteriorates when placed in a dementia-care hospice in accordance with the psychiatrist's advice. Poise and serenity, in fact, are only truly found in the story under study when the 'voice of medicine' (Mishler 1984, 104) is silenced at the story's conclusion and the mother, having regained lucidness, expresses her heartfelt gratitude to Xiangyu for the care conferred upon her over the years, after which the mother is returned to her birth village to die.

Thus, both *Watch for the Happiness* and *Gone is the One Who Held Me Dearest in the World* draw on the prevailing meta-narrative of family caregiving in dementia circulating in Chinese communities, which places day-to-day caregiving duties in the hands of women (Ikels 1998; Zhan 2006). Men play directive but, in the end, largely peripheral roles (Guo 2010). The meta-narrative maintains that women can only be successful in the role if they prioritise their expression of normative Chinese womanhood of 'old' (Croll 1995, 9) over their expression of modernity (Korabik 1993). Both stories posit that modernity need not be wholly erased from the woman's identity, but must be tempered if poise and composure are to be retained and frustration, anger, heartache and self-blame forestalled. This was not voiced in the life stories of family caregiving in dementia analysed in Chapter 5.

The meta-narrative advocates accepting the elderly family member's decline, and the need to care for her or him in the home setting, as normative in old age (Gray *et al.* 2009; Hicks and Lam 1999; Hinton *et al.* 2000; Ikels 2002; Lai and Surood 2009; Liu, D. *et al.* 2008; Wang *et al.* 2006). In the productions discussed in this chapter, biomedicalising the family member's decline as dementia only leads to caregiver self-blame and culpability and untoward outcomes for the person with dementia. This was not voiced in the life story counterparts. The meta-narrative also counsels looking to the past (memory) to sustain the family caregiving endeavour (Holroyd 2001, 2003; Holroyd and Mackenzie 1997). These memories must be of positive experiences from before the onset of illness. Roy (2009) has found in a Canadian literary work dealing with family caregiving in dementia that a wife's memory of past violent behaviour by her ill husband is selectively drawn on to rationalise her decision to institutionalise the husband, despite her deep feelings of love for him. This is a memory, however, of an experience that occurred *after* the onset of illness.

This meta-narrative is drawn on in the productions under study irrespective of the gender of the director. Ma Xiaoying's confident, successful, 'new urban' Chinese woman in *Gone is the One Who Held Me Dearest in the World* does differ from Zeng Xiaoxin's more 'mainstream' modern Chinese woman in *Watch for the Happiness*, possibly because Ma is a woman and Zeng is a man. Yet, both the daughter and daughter-in-law's stories in the two productions endorse the meta-narrative. This is accomplished through the daughter's frequent contravention of this meta-narrative in Ma's film only bringing her regret, frustration, anger and heartache, while the daughter-in-law's broad compliance with this meta-narrative in Zeng's television drama bringing her moral approbation and solace. Thus, a meta-narrative that harks back to a normative Chinese womanhood of 'old' (Croll 1995, 9), in the end, remains largely uncontested in these contemporary productions. This occurs even with a woman director. This indicates the strength of the cultural resonance of the meta-narrative in question.

Conclusion

Analysis of the filmic stories of the experiences of Chinese people caring for a family member with dementia has documented how culture shapes the temporal and causal ordering of life events, the identities claimed and refashioned, and the language used in the stories. As in the life story counterparts analysed in Chapter 5, family caregiving in the filmic stories under study is more readily sustained by looking to the past (indebtedness through memory of the embodied person before illness) rather than to the future (remedy through biomedical intervention). Biomedicine, thus, loses a measure of explanatory value, providing a name for the observed decline in the elderly family member while failing to provide any effective remedial intervention. In contrast, biomedical intervention often proves to be detrimental to both the person with dementia and the family caregiver. At times, biomedical naming is also conflated, in a derogatory sense (Liu, D. *et al.* 2008), with 'madness', reflecting Chinese cultural stigma (see Chapters 2, 3, 4 and 5). Palliation by way of the 'child' metaphor, as voiced in the life story counterparts, is not in evidence in the filmic stories under study, although normalisation by way of old age is implied. Also, as distinct from the life story counterparts, family caregiving in dementia in the filmic stories is decidedly feminised. This feminisation is in line with a normative Chinese womanhood of 'old' (Croll 1995, 9). Overall, a culturally resonant meta-narrative that feminises and normalises family caregiving in dementia is seemingly endorsed by both productions. This occurs regardless of the gender of the director or the form of media production, namely, film and television serial drama.

In sum, this chapter's analysis of filmic stories of family caregiving in dementia complements the analysis of the life stories undertaken in Chapter 5. Analysis of the filmic stories has identified culturally shaped elements unvoiced in the life stories. Cumulatively, they provide insight into how culture shapes Chinese people's stories of family caregiving in dementia told from both inside and outside of the experience.

7 Conclusion

Chapters 2 to 6 have analysed how culture shapes stories of Chinese people's experiences of serious mental illness and family caregiving in dementia. Following the theoretical discussion undertaken in Chapter 1, analytic attention was directed in later chapters to the temporal and causal ordering of life events, the claiming and refashioning of identities, and language use in the stories. These narrative processes, which function to make sense of the illness experience, are interrelated and interconnected (Elliott 2005) and this has been borne out in the preceding analysis.

The onset of mental illness and dementia usually marks a temporal juncture in the lives represented and constructed in the life stories and filmic stories under study. This temporal juncture produces differing levels of 'biographical disruption' (Bury 1982, 169), depending on the illness. The intense stigma toward mental illness in Chinese culture accentuates the level of disruption described in the life stories of family caregiving in mental illness, while a life expectation to care for family members in their old age, instilled through the cultural value of filial piety or a modern adaptation thereof, tempers the level of disruption described in the dementia counterparts. Temporally, the gazes of the life stories and filmic stories discussed in this book also tend to be directed to the past, to before the onset of illness. The life stories of people with a mental illness and their family caregivers look to the recovery of an embodied, social functioning person from before mental illness (Kleinman *et al.* 2011; Traphagan 2000), in accordance with Chinese cultural understandings of recovery. In these stories, the parents of adult-children with a mental illness also draw on their pasts as child-rearers in order to reconcile their cultural obligation to give care at any cost. In the filmic counterparts, the origins of mental illness, too, are unambiguously located in the past, at birth. Cultural stigma sets the cause (blame) for mental illness in heredity. In the life stories and filmic stories of family caregiving in dementia, the cultural value of reciprocity commonly leads to family caregivers reviving positive memories of the embodied person from before in order to sustain caregiving for the now disembodied person in illness. Analysis of the filmic stories found that looking to the future in family caregiving in dementia only brings grief, anger, frustration and heartache.

Identities in the life stories and filmic stories under study are predominantly informed by the past and by cultural forces that stem from tradition. There are few instances of people developing enduring 'new' senses of self, in contrast to the identities claimed and refashioned in Western counterparts (Bury 2001; Frank 1998; Hawkins 1999; Hydén 1997; Riessman 2004). An absence of clear resolution in the life stories of family caregiving in mental illness leads caregivers to seek out meaning by way of their pasts: revisiting and reaffirming culturally valued identities and roles that they had previously enacted (Charon 2006; Hydén 1997). Culture also commonly shapes the life stories of family caregiving in dementia in a way that results in the past (embodied) and the present (disembodied) identities of the person being cared for coexisting contemporaneously. The past identity of the person being cared for is romanticised and gendered in line with Chinese cultural norms. In like manner, normative womanhood in Chinese culture informs the identities claimed and refashioned by women caregivers in the filmic stories of family caregiving in dementia. In these stories, successful family caregiving in dementia requires prioritisation of expression of the normative Chinese womanhood of 'old' over that of 'new' modern Chinese womanhood (Croll 1995). Only in this way can the woman caregiver preserve her moral standing. Such an identity, however, is unsustainable in the filmic stories of women with a mental illness, where attempts to meet the cultural expectations of normative womanhood of 'old' inevitably fail, with the only viable identity in mental illness being that of stigmatised 'other' (Harper 2004).

In the life stores of people with a mental illness, an illness identity, while potentially stigmatising, is able to connect people with a mental illness to a community of fellow sufferers. This imagined community serves as a source of support for the person with a mental illness, while fulfilling a cultural need for connection to others. Claiming an illness identity also allows the person with a mental illness to reconcile the cultural disembodiment experienced in mental illness. Being ill can exonerate, at least amongst family members, the person's inability to fulfil culturally prescribed roles (Hunt 2000; Kleinman 1982). This illness identity, nevertheless, needs to be kept hidden from 'outsiders', due to the intense stigma against mental illness in Chinese culture (Kleinman *et al.* 2011; Lam *et al.* 2011).[1]

The language of battle, a common feature of Western illness stories, is employed in formulaic ways in the life stories of people with a mental illness and their family caregivers. All three elements that Hawkins (1999) posits are necessary for the effective expression of the battle metaphor in illness are present in these stories: an identified enemy (mental illness); an alliance with the health professional (working 'hand-in-hand' with the psychiatrist and psychologist); and the use of therapeutic weaponry (psychotropic medication). The battle metaphor employed in these life stories, nevertheless, retains a historical and political resonance that culturally binds it to mainland China. At the same time, the use of the battle metaphor in these stories encapsulates the effort required to meet the cultural expectation to return a person with mental illness to her or his former embodied state and fully contribute to society through work or study. Immense differences in levels of social functioning separate the cultural expectation from the reality of the illness condition.

In addition to the language of battle, natural calamities familiar to the 'everyday world' (Hydén 1995, 73) are figuratively drawn on in the life stories of family caregiving in mental illness to express the profound cultural, economic and emotional burden that family caregivers and their families shoulder in mental illness. The added intensity of tragedy expressed through the use of such a metaphor finds explanation in the acute stigma against mental illness in Chinese culture. This stigma expands beyond the afflicted individual to seriously taint healthy family members and damage their social and cultural standing ('face') (Ramsay 2008). Future marriage prospects, for example, are jeopardised. This is because an essential element of Chinese cultural stigma is mental illness's deemed pollution of family blood lines. This manifests in the filmic stories of people with a mental illness through conspicuous linguistic references to birth and family names.

Chinese cultural stigma also shapes the life stories and filmic stories of mental illness through a figurative depiction of people with a mental illness as 'trash'. In like manner, some of the life stories and filmic stories of family caregiving in dementia display a pejorative use of the vocabulary of mental illness [疯子; 疯妈] and of dementia [老人痴呆症]. This is linked in these stories to people's biomedicalisation of dementia. Most of the life stories of family caregiving in dementia, however, normalise the signs of dementia as simply old age. These stories figuratively engage the 'child' metaphor, the use of which, it is argued, is shaped by a cultural script that states that, toward the end of life, a Chinese person will typically 'return to a childlike state' (Hinton *et al.* 2000, 125).

The above-mentioned connection between the use of pejorative language in the life stories and filmic stories of family caregiving in dementia and the biomedicalisation of dementia by people in these stories points to the potential intersection between a biomedical aetiological explanation of dementia, which can allude to genetic factors, and Chinese cultural stigma grounded in heredity (Hinton *et al.* 2000). This intersection also explains the silencing of the biomedical aetiological explanation in the life stories of family caregiving in dementia, where preference is given to normalising the signs of dementia as simply old age. This occurs despite visits to health professionals frequently featuring in these stories. In like manner, the potential intersection between the biomedical aetiological explanation and Chinese cultural stigma grounded in heredity explains the silencing of the biomedical aetiological explanation in the life stories of people with a mental illness, where a less face-threatening psychosocial aetiological explanation is more commonly voiced. This occurs despite the psychoeducational context of publication of the life stories, the authority bestowed upon health professional advice by the person with a mental illness in these stories, and a documented hegemony of the biomedical explanatory model of mental illness in mainland Chinese mental health circles

(Kleinman and Kleinman 1985; Pearson 1995a; Phillips 1993; Ramsay 2008; Ran *et al.* 2005; Tseng 1986).

These findings add weight to Hinton *et al.*'s (2000, 134) claim that, when undertaking dementia research in Chinese populations, 'biomedical labels, even though they are employed with good intentions, may be very stigmatizing and have negative impact within the participants' cultural context.' This would equally apply to the use of such labels in clinical settings where services are provided to Chinese clients. Other findings of this book which may be of value in the clinical environment include awareness that the notions of stigma and recovery, while seemingly culturally transposable, are, in fact, highly shaped by Chinese cultural understandings, for example, of disease aetiology and the normative life pathway. Marginalisation of people with a mental illness may be a universal phenomenon, however, analysis of the life stories and filmic stories of mental illness and identification of the prevailing meta-narrative circulating in Chinese communities demonstrate the extent to which, in Chinese culture, this can be traced to a deemed tainted genetic makeup. Similarly, notions of success and recovery in mental illness can stem from a decidedly gendered, Chinese cultural prescription of social functioning, rather than from individually-derived measures of achievement (Ng *et al.* 2011, 2012).

Clinicians may also find benefit in knowing that stories told by family caregivers in mental illness at clinical interview may seek to draw attention to an observance of Chinese cultural prescriptions to give care at all costs, which becomes the 'fundamental moral challenge' in family caregiving in mental illness (Hydén 1995, 67), and to fully comply with health professional advice. At the same time, they may refrain from drawing attention to personal gains obtained through positive reinterpretation of the family caregiving endeavour or through ongoing renegotiation of the family caregiving role. While likely seen as unremarkable in Western stories of family caregiving in mental illness, accounts of personal gain could be construed as culturally transgressive in Chinese counterparts. Clinicians may also need to be mindful that the telling of these 'heroic' tales of self-sacrifice, figuratively steeped in notions of battle and natural calamity, may, in the end, be detrimental in placing an immense burden of cultural expectation on the family caregiver, which she or he is possibly unable to meet (Couser 1997, 45). The culturally prescribed end-goals in recovery, namely, holding down a job or studies, being productive in the workforce and meeting the norms of social interaction, remain problematic in mental illness (Ng *et al.* 2008b). This is brought out in the life stories analysed in Chapters 2 and 3. This is also unambiguously stated in the filmic counterparts and in the meta-narrative of mental illness they affirm. Unattainability of the culturally prescribed end-goals in recovery could, over the longer term, serve as an intense source of frustration for the family caregiver, whose non-negotiable cultural obligation is to ensure that these end-goals are reached. A danger, as borne out in a number of the life stories and filmic stories of mental illness under study, is that the family caregiver may choose to vent her or his frustration in a detrimental (violent) way or to abandon the family caregiving enterprise altogether.

As to clients who are family caregiving in dementia, clinicians may find benefit in knowing that the clients' revival of positive memories of the person before illness may sustain their motivation in the family caregiving endeavour by meeting an essential condition for expression of the Chinese cultural value of reciprocity (Holroyd 2001, 2003; Holroyd and Mackenzie 1997). Clinicians may also benefit from being aware of the culturally derived reluctance to biomedicalise dementia and the cultural resonance of the 'child' metaphor in family caregiving in dementia. Clinicians may also wish to take note of the prevailing meta-narrative of family caregiving in dementia disseminated by Chinese popular media such as film and television serial drama. A somewhat disempowering meta-narrative identified in this book feminises family caregiving in dementia, in a way that problematicises notions of modern Chinese womanhood (Cook and Dong 2011; Croll 1995; Guo 2010; Kong 2008; Korabik 1993; Mann 2011).

A strength of this book lies in its use of life stories and filmic stories as complementary data sources (Brody 2003; Hydén 1997; Lieblich *et al.* 1998; Lupton 2003; Toolan 2001). This has allowed examination of how Chinese culture shapes accounts of mental illness and accounts of dementia which have been proffered by those inside and outside of the experience. It has also allowed culturally shaped narrative continuities and departures to be identified, with filmic accounts commonly giving voice to what remains unvoiced in life accounts (Beck *et al.* 2005; Harter *et al.* 2005; Kirmayer 2000; Riessman 1993; Squire 2005). Through examination of filmic stories, the relevant prevailing meta-narratives circulating in Chinese communities and drawn on by popular media such as film and television serial drama have been more singularly identified. These have been shown to 'articulate and reproduce existing ideologies and hegemonic relations of power and inequality' (Ewick and Silbey, quoted in Elliott 2005, 146), both in mental illness (stigmatisation and marginalisation) and in family caregiving in dementia (feminisation of caregiving and problematicisation of modern Chinese womanhood). Examination of the life stories, on the other hand, has revealed how culture shapes these stories in ways that both disempower *and* reassure in mental illness and in family caregiving in dementia. Cultural norms and scripts dictate and constrain behaviours and responses as well as cede authority to health professionals where diagnoses are not in dispute. Cultural values and understandings result in the (embodied) person from before illness being valued over the (disembodied) person of now. At the same time, cultural understandings, norms, values and scripts offer comfort and solace in mental illness and in family caregiving in dementia, by imparting senses of certainty, familiarity and continuity amidst the challenges faced.

As stated at the outset of this book, the potential for alternative readings of illness stories as data remains a hallmark of research such as that undertaken in the book (Clandinin and Connelly 2000; Clandinin and Rosiek 2007; Freeman 2001; Lieblich *et al.* 1998; Lupton 2003; Riessman 2000). While culture constitutes a central concern of this book, other disciplinary perspectives may provide distinct yet equally insightful interpretations of the data in question. Gender, most notably, has emerged as an important issue in the current data. Future research, therefore, may wish to further examine Chinese life stories and filmic stories of mental illness and family caregiving in dementia by making use of the theoretical perspectives and analytic approaches offered by gender studies (Bengs *et al.* 2008; Charteris-Black and Seale 2010; Emslie *et al.* 2006; Galasiński 2008; Hequembourg and Brallier 2005). This would provide 'greater attention to ways in which gender matters in the cultural narratives about being mad' (Chouinard 2009, 803) than was possible given the scope of this book.

We have explored how 'culturally based understandings shape or are reflected in stories about specific, often very personal, experiences with illness' (Garro and Mattingly 2000a, 28). This has been achieved, it is believed, through bringing together, in a structured and transparent way, individual findings from analyses of life stories and filmic stories about mental illness and family caregiving in dementia. The book's findings bear out the important role that culture plays in shaping stories such as those under study. It is hoped that this is of benefit to those engaged in the academic study of culture, illness and story; and of Chinese society more broadly. It is also hoped that this is of benefit to those whose professional and personal responsibilities, across the globe, bring them into contact with Chinese people facing mental illness and family caregiving in dementia (Blignault *et al.* 2008; Hurwitz *et al.* 2004; Kleinman *et al.* 2006; Riessman 2004; Skultans 2003).

Notes

1 Introduction

1 Following Garro and Mattingly (2000a, 2000b), Squire (2005) and Thornborrow and Coates (2005), this book does not distinguish between the expressions 'narrative' and 'story', as some researchers do. There is no common agreement on this distinction, and the distinction, for the most part, does not fundamentally engage this book's exploration of how culture shapes the life stories and filmic stories under study. As a consequence, the two expressions are considered interchangeable throughout this book.

2 Life stories of people with a mental illness

1 Translation of the original bibliographic information from Chinese [in the square brackets] into English is the work of the book's author.
2 For terminological convenience, the qualifier *personal* is used hereafter to refer to life stories authored by people with a mental illness (as opposed to their family caregivers, whose life stories are analysed in Chapter 3).
3 Data examples are presented in the format of English translation first followed by the original Chinese source text [in the square brackets] and its citation. All translations are the work of the book's author, unless otherwise indicated. Riessman (2000) has noted that translating adds yet another interpretative level to the analysis of such stories, which already constitutes a researcher's interpretation of a storyteller's interpretation of events (see Chapter 1). In order to minimise the effects of this 'third' level of interpretation, the translations in this book are rendered as faithful as possible to the original source text while maintaining a reasonable degree of English language idiomaticity.
4 One Yuan is approximately fifteen US cents.
5 One Jiao is approximately one and a half US cents.
6 Many thanks to the anonymous reviewer for this insight.
7 Most people with a mental illness in mainland China do not have access to rehabilitation facilities (Yip 2007).
8 Research undertaken in Hong Kong by Ng *et al.* (2008a, 2008b, 2011) involving Chinese people with a mental illness and Chinese practicing and trainee mental health professionals identifies similar 'social' criteria for defining recovery (Ng *et al.* 2011, 249), along with an absence of relapse and a cessation of medication. Ng *et al.* (2011, 258) consider that such a definition of recovery is '[a]uthoritative, paternalistic' and 'mythical' and ultimately 'detrimental to [mental health service] users in collectivist societies, such as the Chinese'.

9　Further details about psychoeducational programs in mainland China are reported in Xiang, Ran and Li (1994), Xiong *et al.* (1994), Yip (2005), Zhang *et al.* (1993) and Zhang *et al.* (1994).

10　In contrast to the positive assessments made in the life stories analysed in the current chapter, the family caregiver counterparts analysed in Chapter 3 *do* foreground the obstacles to recovery that broader society commonly presents. It is argued in Chapter 3 that such a narrative position reinforces the *family caregivers'* principal cultural duty to resolutely give care in the face of all obstacles.

11　It should be noted that most people with a mental illness in mainland China do not have access to psychiatrists and psychologists (Yip 2007).

12　Regret over initially seeking out spiritual healers, and, so, delaying presentation to formal health services, is expressed in the family caregiver counterparts analysed in Chapter 3.

3　Life stories of family caregiving in mental illness

1　Parts of this chapter are drawn from Ramsay, 2010, Mainland Chinese family caregiver narratives in mental illness: disruption and continuity, *Asian Studies Review*, volume 34, pages 83–103. The author thanks Taylor & Francis Ltd, http://www.tandf.co.uk/journals, for permitting publication of the content in this book.

2　Pearson and Lam (2002, 174) have found in their mainland Chinese (Guangzhou) study that '[f]amilies were quite speedy in seeking treatment for their relatives after the first onset' of mental illness, 'with 31 per cent consulting some kind of psychiatric service within the first month', rising to 90 per cent within a year of onset. They do note, however, that such a finding 'contravenes the commonly held view … that Chinese families delay seeking help beyond the confines of relatives and trusted outsiders for as long as possible, sometimes for years' (174). It should be noted that, in addition to families' inability to recognise symptoms or their fear of public disclosure when symptoms are recognised, delayed presentation can commonly result from unavailability of or lack of knowledge of appropriate mental health services as well as their frequently prohibitive cost (Yip 2007).

3　Kleinman (1988, 20) observes that, in Chinese societies, the diagnosis '"neurasthenia" … provides a legitimate physical disease label as a cloak to disguise psychiatric problems that remain illegitimate and unacceptable.'

4　That Anding Hospital is one of the best and most expensive psychiatric hospitals in mainland China signifies the extraordinary effort and cost afforded by this family caregiver. Many thanks to the anonymous reviewer for this insight.

5　One Yuan is approximately fifteen US cents.

6　One Jiao is approximately one and a half US cents.

7　Face is a cultural phenomenon denoting concern for 'how one is evaluated by others' (Hinze 2002, 269). Face lies at the heart of Confucian teachings on social and interpersonal relationships and, as such, maintains a high degree of salience in social and 'moral' behaviour in Confucian-heritage societies like mainland China (Wong 2000; Yang and Kleinman 2008).

8　The expression 'for historical reasons' [由于历史的原因] is a commonly-used mainland Chinese expression, particularly in political discourse, alluding to unspecified causative factors from the past which remain beyond the control of the speaker.

9　Phillips *et al.* (2002, 488) call for greater clinical attention to individual emotional responses and reactions to cultural stigma in mental illness, stating that 'the most damaging effect of stigma and discrimination is the subjective internalisation of these negative valuations.'

5   Life stories of family caregiving in dementia

1   Thanks also to the anonymous reviewer for this insight.
2   While 'dementia' or 'senility' are linguistically more correct translations of 老年痴呆症, here 'Alzheimer's disease' is used, following the practice used in the official English language title of the Hong Kong Alzheimer's Disease Association.
3   Hereafter, HKADAPG.
4   This is the English language title employed in the book.
5   This is the English language name employed in the book.
6   It should be noted that elsewhere in Lee's (2005) story of family caregiving in dementia his wife's personhood in illness is also warmly honoured.
7   While the expression 痴呆症 (containing 痴呆, which literally means 'stupid/retarded') has been retained in formal settings in Hong Kong and mainland China, its pejorative use has seen it replaced in formal settings in Taiwan by a more neutral expression 失智症 (containing 失智, which literally means 'loss of intellect/reasoning'). Less commonly, a transliteration of the English expression 'Alzheimer's disease' [阿爾茨海默氏症] also appears in biomedically informed settings across all regions.

6   Filmic stories of family caregiving in dementia

1   It is common for Chinese cinematic productions to be adaptations of published literary works (Deppman 2010).
2   Hinton *et al.* (2000, 130) state that Chinese cultural stigma manifests in dementia

> '[a]t the point when an older person loses their social awareness [and] cross[es] the line separating "normal" age-related memory loss from pathological, "crazy" memory loss.' Ascribing the 'mad' label results in 'Alzheimer's disease, like severe mental illness, … [being] perceived as an inherited family condition, which, if known by the greater community, can decrease the marriage prospects of younger family members' (Hinton *et al.* 2000, 130).

7   Conclusion

1   Lam *et al.* (2011, 584) state that in Hong Kong 'It is not uncommon in psychiatric clinical practice for patients to ask for a "fake" diagnosis and the use of non-psychiatric hospital stamps on sick leave certificates in an attempt to conceal the illness.'

References

Au, A., Lai, M. K., Lau, K. M., Pan, P. C., Lam, L., Thompson, L. and Gallagher-Thompson, D. 2009. Social support and well-being in dementia family caregivers: the mediating role of self-efficacy. *Aging and Mental Health*, 13 (5), 761–768.

Au, A., Li, S., Lee, K., Leung, P., Pan, P. C., Thompson, L. and Gallagher-Thompson, D. 2010. The Coping with Caregiving group program for Chinese caregivers of patients with Alzheimer's disease in Hong Kong. *Patient Education and Counseling*, 78, 256–260.

Ayometzi, C. C. 2007. Storying as becoming: identity through the telling of conversion. In M. Bamberg, A. De Fina and D. Schiffrin (eds) *Selves and identities in narrative and discourse* (pp. 41–70). Amsterdam: John Benjamins.

Babrow, A. S., Kline, K. N. and Rawlins, W. K. 2005. Narrating problems and problematizing narratives: linking problematic integration and narrative theory in telling stories about our health. In L. M. Harter, P. M. Japp and C. S. Beck (eds) *Narratives, health, and healing: communication theory, research, and practice* (pp. 31–52). Mahwah, NJ, US: L. Erlbaum Associates.

Bahl, V. 1999. Mental illness: a national perspective. In D. Bhugra and V. Bahl (eds) *Ethnicity: an agenda for mental health* (pp. 7–22). London: Gaskell/The Royal College of Psychiatrists.

Bakhtin, M. M. 1981. *The dialogic imagination: four essays*. Austin, TX, US: University of Texas Press.

Bakken, B. 2000. *The exemplary society: human improvement, social control, and the dangers of modernity in China*. Oxford, UK: Oxford University Press.

Bamberg, M., De Fina, A. and Schiffrin, D. 2007. Introduction. In M. Bamberg, A. De Fina and D. Schiffrin (eds) *Selves and identities in narrative and discourse* (pp. 1–8). Amsterdam: John Benjamins.

Barrett, R. 1996. *The psychiatric team and the social definition of schizophrenia: an anthropological study of person and illness*. Cambridge, UK: Cambridge University Press.

Bartlett, M. C., Gorman, J., Brauner, D. J., Graham, M. E., Coats, B. C., Marder, R., England, S. E., Miller, B., Gaibel, L., O'Shea, B., Ganzer, C. and Poirier, S. 1993. Moral reasoning and Alzheimer's care: exploring complex weavings through narrative. *Journal of Aging Studies*, 7 (4), 409–421.

Beck, C. S., Harter, L. M. and Japp, P. M. 2005. Afterword: continuing the conversation: reflections on our emergent scholarly narratives. In L. M. Harter, P. M. Japp and C. S. Beck (eds) *Narratives, health, and healing: communication theory, research, and practice* (pp. 433–444). Mahwah, NJ, US: L. Erlbaum Associates.

Bengs, C., Johansson, E., Danielsson, U., Lehti, A. and Hammarström, A. 2008. Gendered portraits of depression in Swedish newspapers. *Qualitative Health Research*, 18 (7), 962–973.

Bentelspacher, C. E., Chitran, S. and Rahman, M. B. A. 1994. Coping and adaptation patterns among Chinese, Indian, and Malay families caring for a mentally ill relative. *Families in Society*, 75 (5), 287–294.

Berger, A. A. 1997. *Narratives in popular culture, media, and everyday life.* Thousand Oaks, CA, US: Sage.

Bhugra, D. 2006. *Mad tales from Bollywood: portrayal of mental illness in conventional Hindi cinema.* New York: Psychology Press.

Biegel, D. E., Sales, E. and Schulz, R. 1991. *Family caregiving in chronic illness: Alzheimer's disease, cancer, heart disease, mental illness, and stroke.* Newbury Park, CA, US: Sage.

Birch, M. 2012. *Mediating mental health: contexts, debates and analysis.* Farnham, UK: Ashgate Publishing.

Blignault, I., Ponzio, V., Rong, Y. and Eisenbruch, M. 2008. A qualitative study of barriers to mental health services utilisation among migrants from mainland China in south-east Sydney. *International Journal of Social Psychiatry*, 54 (2), 180–190.

Bordwell, D. 1985. *Narration in the fiction film.* Madison, WI, US: University of Wisconsin Press.

Branigan, E. 1992. *Narrative comprehension and film.* London: Routledge.

Brassington, C. 1995. *The portrayal of disability in contemporary Chinese literature and its relationship to perceptions of and attitudes towards people with disabilities in contemporary Chinese society: an investigative study.* Unpublished doctoral dissertation. St Lucia, QLD, Australia: The University of Queensland.

Braun, K. L. and Browne, C. V. 1998. Perceptions of dementia, caregiving, and help seeking among Asian and Pacific Islander Americans. *Health and Social Work*, 23 (4), 262–274.

Brockmeier, J. and Carbaugh, D. 2001. Introduction. In J. Brockmeier and D. Carbaugh (eds) *Narrative and identity: studies in autobiography, self and culture* (pp. 1–24). Amsterdam: John Benjamins.

Brody, H. 2003. *Stories of sickness.* Oxford, UK: Oxford University Press.

Brown, J. W. and Alligood, M. R. 2004. Realizing wrongness: stories of older wife caregivers. *The Journal of Applied Gerontology*, 23 (2), 104–119.

Bury, M. 1982. Chronic illness as biographical disruption. *Sociology of Health and Illness*, 4 (2), 167–182.

Bury, M. 2001. Illness narratives: fact or fiction? *Sociology of Health and Illness*, 23 (3), 263–285.

Callan, A. and Littlewood, R. 1998. Patient satisfaction: ethnic origin or explanatory model? *International Journal of Social Psychiatry*, 44 (1), 1–11.

Carabas, T. and Harter, L. M. 2005. State-induced illness and forbidden stories: the role of storytelling in healing individual and social traumas in Romania. In L. M. Harter, P. M. Japp and C. S. Beck (eds) *Narratives, health, and healing: communication theory, research, and practice* (pp. 149–168). Mahwah, NJ, US: L. Erlbaum Associates.

Carney, S. 2004. Transcendent stories and counternarratives in holocaust survivor life histories: searching for meaning in video-testimony archives. In C. Daiute and C. Lightfoot (eds) *Narrative analysis: studying the development of individuals in society* (pp. 201–222). Thousand Oaks, CA, US: Sage.

Charon, R. 2006. *Narrative medicine: honoring the stories of illness.* Oxford, UK: Oxford University Press.

Charteris-Black, J. and Seale, C. 2010. *Gender and the language of illness.* Basingstoke, UK: Palgrave Macmillan.

Cheng, S. T. 2009. The social networks of nursing-home residents in Hong Kong. *Ageing and Society*, 29, 163–178.

Cheshire, J. and Ziebland, S. 2005. Narrative as a resource in accounts of the experience of illness. In J. Thornborrow and J. Coates (eds) *The sociolinguistics of narrative* (pp. 17–40). Amsterdam: John Benjamins.

Cheung, C. K. and Kwan, A. Y. H. 2009. The erosion of filial piety by modernisation in Chinese cities. *Ageing and Society*, 29, 179–198.

Chouinard, V. 2009. Placing the 'mad woman': troubling cultural representations of being a woman with mental illness in *Girl, Interrupted. Social and Cultural Geography*, 10 (7), 791–804.

Chow, N. 1990. Ageing in Hong Kong. In B. K. P. Leung (ed.) *Social issues in Hong Kong* (pp. 164–177). Hong Kong: Oxford University Press.

Chow, N. W. S. 2001. The practice of filial piety among the Chinese in Hong Kong. In I. Chi, N. L. Chappell and J. Lubben (eds) *Elderly Chinese in Pacific rim countries: social support and integration* (pp. 125–136). Hong Kong: Hong Kong University Press.

Chung, J. C. C. 2001. Empowering individuals with early dementia and their carers: an exploratory study in the Chinese context. *American Journal of Alzheimer's Disease and Other Dementias*, 16 (2), 85–88.

Clandinin, D. J. and Connelly, F. M. 2000. *Narrative inquiry: experience and story in qualitative research.* San Francisco, CA, US: Jossey-Bass Inc.

Clandinin, D. J. and Rosiek, J. 2007. Mapping a landscape of narrative inquiry: borderland spaces and tensions. In D. J. Clandinin (ed.) *Handbook of narrative inquiry: mapping a methodology* (pp. 35–76). Thousand Oaks, CA, US: Sage.

Cohen, L. 1998. *No aging in India: Alzheimer's, the bad family, and other modern things.* Berkeley, US: University of California Press.

Cook, S. and Dong, X. Y. 2011. Harsh choices: Chinese women's paid work and unpaid care responsibilities under economic reform. *Development and Change*, 42 (4), 947–965.

Cora-Bramble, D. and Williams, L. 2000. Explaining illness to Latinos: cultural foundations and messages. In B. B. Whaley (ed.) *Explaining illness: research, theory, and strategies* (pp. 249–270). Mahwah, NJ, US: Lawrence Erlbaum Associates.

Cortazzi, M. 1993. *Narrative analysis.* London: Falmer Press.

Couser, G. T. 1997. *Recovering bodies: illness, disability, and life-writing.* Madison, WI, US: University of Wisconsin Press.

Croll, E. 1995. *Changing identities of Chinese women: rhetoric, experience and self-perception in twentieth century China.* Hong Kong: Hong Kong University Press.

Daiute, C. and Lightfoot, C. 2004. Editors' introduction: theory and craft in narrative inquiry. In C. Daiute and C. Lightfoot (eds) *Narrative analysis: studying the development of individuals in society* (pp. vii–xviii). Thousand Oaks, CA, US: Sage.

Deppman, H. C. 2010. *Adapted for the screen: the cultural politics of adaptation in modern Chinese fiction and film.* Honolulu: University of Hawaii Press.

Dikötter, F. 1998. *Imperfect conceptions: medical knowledge, birth defects and eugenics in China.* London: Hurst & Co.

Elliott, J. 2005. *Using narrative in social research: qualitative and quantitative approaches*. Thousand Oaks, CA, US: Sage.

Emslie, C., Ridge, D., Ziebland, S. and Hunt, K. 2006. Men's accounts of depression: reconstructing or resisting hegemonic masculinity? *Social Science and Medicine*, 62, 2246–2257.

Fan, C. and Karnilowicz, W. 2000. Attitudes towards mental illness and knowledge of mental health services among the Australian and Chinese community. *Australian Journal of Primary Health*, 6 (2), 38–48.

Feldman, C. F. 2001. Narratives of national identity as group narratives: patterns of interpretive cognition. In J. Brockmeier and D. Carbaugh (eds) *Narrative and identity: studies in autobiography, self and culture* (pp. 129–144). Amsterdam: John Benjamins.

Feng, L., Chiu, H., Chong, M. Y., Yu, X. and Kua, E. H. 2011. Dementia in Chinese populations: current data and future research. *Asia-Pacific Psychiatry*, 3 (3), 109–114.

Frank, A. W. 1995. *The wounded storyteller: body, illness, and ethics*. Chicago, US: University of Chicago Press.

Frank, A. W. 1998. Just listening: narrative and deep illness. *Families, Systems and Health*, 16 (3), 197–212.

Frank, A. W. 2009. The necessity and dangers of illness narratives, especially at the end of life. In Y. Gunaratnam and D. Oliviere (eds) *Narrative and stories in health care: illness, dying, and bereavement* (pp. 161–176). Oxford, UK: Oxford University Press.

Frank, A. W. 2010. *Letting stories breathe: a socio-narratology*. Chicago, US: University of Chicago Press.

Freeman, M. 2001. From substance to story: narrative, identity, and the reconstruction of the self. In J. Brockmeier and D. Carbaugh (eds) *Narrative and identity: studies in autobiography, self and culture* (pp. 283–298). Amsterdam: John Benjamins.

Freeman, M. 2004. Data are everywhere: narrative criticism in the literature of experience. In C. Daiute and C. Lightfoot (eds) *Narrative analysis: studying the development of individuals in society* (pp. 63–82). Thousand Oaks, CA, US: Sage.

Fuery, P. 2003. *Madness and cinema: psychoanalysis, spectatorship, and culture*. New York: Palgrave Macmillan.

Gabriel, Y. 2004. The voice of experience and the voice of the expert – can they speak to each other? In B. Hurwitz, T. Greenhalgh and V. Skultans (eds) *Narrative research in health and illness* (pp. 168–186). Malden, MA, US: BMJ Books.

Galasiński, D. 2008. *Men's discourses of depression*. New York: Palgrave Macmillan.

Gallagher-Thompson, D., Wang, P. C., Liu, W., Cheung, V., Peng, R., China, D. and Thompson, L. W. 2010. Effectiveness of a psychoeducational skill training DVD program to reduce stress in Chinese American dementia caregivers: results of a preliminary study. *Aging and Mental Health*, 14 (3), 263–273.

Garden, R. 2010. Telling stories about illness and disability: the limits and lessons of narrative. *Perspectives in Biology and Medicine*, 53 (1), 121–135.

Garro, L. C. 2000. Cultural knowledge as resource in illness narratives: remembering through accounts of illness. In C. Mattingly and L. C. Garro (eds) *Narrative and the cultural construction of illness and healing* (pp. 70–87). Berkeley, US: University of California Press.

Garro, L. C. 2001. The remembered past in a culturally meaningful life: remembering as cultural, social, and cognitive process. In C. C. Moore and H. F. Mathews (eds) *The psychology of cultural experience* (pp. 105–147). Cambridge, UK: Cambridge University Press.

Garro, L. C. and Mattingly, C. 2000a. Narrative as construct and as construction. In C. Mattingly and L. C. Garro (eds) *Narrative and the cultural construction of illness and healing* (pp. 1–49). Berkeley, US: University of California Press.

Garro, L. C. and Mattingly, C. 2000b. Narrative turns. In C. Mattingly and L. C. Garro (eds) *Narrative and the cultural construction of illness and healing* (pp. 259–270). Berkeley, US: University of California Press.

Gergen, M. 2004. Once upon a time: a narratologist's tale. In C. Daiute and C. Lightfoot (eds) *Narrative analysis: studying the development of individuals in society* (pp. 267–286). Thousand Oaks, CA, US: Sage.

Glick, D. and Applbaum, K. 2010. Dangerous noncompliance: a narrative analysis of a CNN special investigation of mental illness. *Anthropology and Medicine*, 17 (2), 229–244.

Good, B. J. and Good, M. J. D. 2000. 'Fiction' and 'Historicity' in doctors' stories: social and narrative dimensions of learning medicine. In C. Mattingly and L. C. Garro (eds) *Narrative and the cultural construction of illness and healing* (pp. 50–69). Berkeley, US: University of California Press.

Gray, H. L., Jimenez, D. E., Cucciare, M. A., Tong, H. Q. and Gallagher-Thompson, D. 2009. Ethnic differences in beliefs regarding Alzheimer's disease among dementia family caregivers. *American Journal of Geriatric Psychiatry*, 17 (11), 925–933.

Gui, S. 2001. Care of the elderly in one-child families in China: issues and measures. In I. Chi, N. L. Chappell and J. Lubben (eds) *Elderly Chinese in Pacific rim countries: social support and integration* (pp. 115–124). Hong Kong: Hong Kong University Press.

Guo, Y. 2010. China's celebrity mothers: female virtues, patriotism and social harmony. In L. Edwards and E. Jeffreys (eds) *Celebrity in China* (pp. 45–66). Hong Kong: Hong Kong University Press.

Harden, J. 2005. Parenting a young person with mental health problems: temporal disruption and reconstruction. *Sociology of Health and Illness*, 27 (3), 351–371.

Harper, D. J. 2004. Storying policy: constructions of risk in proposals to reform UK mental health legislation. In B. Hurwitz, T. Greenhalgh and V. Skultans (eds) *Narrative research in health and illness* (pp. 397–413). Malden, MA, US: BMJ Books.

Harter, L. M., Japp, P. M. and Beck, C. S. 2005. Vital problematics of narrative theorizing about health and healing. In L. M. Harter, P. M. Japp and C. S. Beck (eds) *Narratives, health, and healing: communication theory, research, and practice* (pp. 7–30). Mahwah, NJ, US: L. Erlbaum Associates.

Hawkins, A. H. 1999. *Reconstructing illness: studies in pathography* (2nd edn). West Lafayette, IN, US: Purdue University Press.

Hayne, Y. and Yonge, O. 1997. The lifeworld of the chronic mentally ill: analysis of 40 written personal accounts. *Archives of Psychiatric Nursing*, XI (6), 314–324.

Hemsley, B., Balandin, S. and Togher, L. 2007. Narrative analysis of the hospital experience for older parents of people who cannot speak. *Journal of Aging Studies*, 21, 239–254.

Hequembourg, A. and Brallier, S. 2005. Gendered stories of parental caregiving among siblings. *Journal of Aging Studies*, 19, 53–71.

Hicks, M. H. R. and Lam, M. S. C. 1999. Decision-making within the social course of dementia: accounts by Chinese-American caregivers. *Culture, Medicine and Psychiatry*, 23, 415–452.

Hiday, V. A. 1995. The social context of mental illness and violence. *Journal of Health and Social Behavior*, 36 (2), 122–137.

Hinton, L., Guo, Z., Hillygus, J. and Levkoff, S. 2000. Working with culture: a qualitative analysis of barriers to the recruitment of Chinese-American family caregivers for dementia research. *Journal of Cross-Cultural Gerontology*, 15, 119–137.

Hinton, W. L. and Levkoff, S. 1999. Constructing Alzheimer's: narratives of lost identities, confusion and loneliness in old age. *Culture, Medicine and Psychiatry*, 23, 453–475.

Hinze, C. 2002. *Re-thinking 'face': pursuing an emic-etic understanding of Chinese mian and lian and English face*. Unpublished doctoral dissertation. St Lucia, QLD, Australia: The University of Queensland.

Ho, B., Friedland, J., Rappolt, S. and Noh, S. 2003. Caregiving for relatives with Alzheimer's disease: feelings of Chinese-Canadian women. *Journal of Aging Studies*, 17, 301–321.

Holroyd, E. 2001. Hong Kong Chinese daughters' intergenerational caregiving obligations: a cultural model approach. *Social Science and Medicine*, 53, 1125–1134.

Holroyd, E. 2003. Chinese family obligations toward chronically ill elderly members: comparing caregivers in Beijing and Hong Kong. *Qualitative Health Research*, 13 (3), 302–318.

Holroyd, E. and Mackenzie, A. E. 1995. A review of the historical and social processes contributing to care and caregiving in Chinese families. *Journal of Advanced Nursing*, 22, 473–479.

Holroyd, E. and Mackenzie, A. E. 1997. Beijing families: the behavior and sentiment of caregiving. *Journal of Family Nursing*, 3 (4), 348–364.

Hong Kong Alzheimer's Disease Association Publishing Group [香港老年痴呆症協會出版組] (ed.). 2002. 不離不棄: 老年痴呆症患者家屬照顧心聲. 香港: 香港老年痴呆症協會 and 香港復康會社區復康網絡.

Hunt, L. M. 2000. Strategic suffering: illness narratives as social empowerment among Mexican cancer patients. In C. Mattingly and L. C. Garro (eds) *Narrative and the cultural construction of illness and healing* (pp. 88–107). Berkeley, US: University of California Press.

Hurwitz, B. 2004. The temporal construction of medical narratives. In B. Hurwitz, T. Greenhalgh and V. Skultans (eds) *Narrative research in health and illness* (pp. 414–427). Malden, MA, US: BMJ Books.

Hurwitz, B., Greenhalgh, T. and Skultans, V. 2004. Introduction. In B. Hurwitz, T. Greenhalgh and V. Skultans (eds) *Narrative research in health and illness* (pp. 1–20). Malden, MA, US: BMJ Books.

Hydén, L. C. 1995. In search of an ending: narrative reconstruction as a moral quest. *Journal of Narrative and Life History*, 5 (1), 67–84.

Hydén, L. C. 1997. Illness and narrative. *Sociology of Health and Illness*, 19 (1), 48–69.

Hydén, L. C. 2008. Broken and vicarious voices in narratives. In L. C. Hydén and J. Brockmeier (eds) *Health, illness and culture: broken narratives* (pp. 36–53). New York: Routledge.

Hydén, L. C. and Brockmeier, J. 2008. Introduction: from the retold to the performed story. In L. C. Hydén and J. Brockmeier (eds) *Health, illness and culture: broken narratives* (pp. 1–15). New York: Routledge.

Hydén, L. C. and Örulv, L. 2009. Narrative and identity in Alzheimer's disease: a case study. *Journal of Aging Studies*, 23, 205–214.

Ikels, C. 1998. The experience of dementia in China. *Culture, Medicine and Psychiatry*, 22, 257–283.

Ikels, C. 2002. Constructing and deconstructing the self: dementia in China. *Journal of Cross-Cultural Gerontology*, 17, 233–251.

Japp, P. M. 2005. Personal narratives and public dialogues: introduction. In L. M. Harter, P. M. Japp and C. S. Beck (eds) *Narratives, health, and healing: communication theory, research, and practice* (pp. 53–59). Mahwah, NJ, US: L. Erlbaum Associates.

Jones, R. A. 2005. Identity commitments in personal stories of mental illness on the internet. *Narrative Inquiry*, 15 (2), 293–322.

Jones, R. S., Chow, T. W. and Gatz, M. 2006. Asian Americans and Alzheimer's disease: assimilation, culture, and beliefs. *Journal of Aging Studies*, 20, 11–25.

King, A. Y. C. and Bond, M. H. 1985. The Confucian paradigm of man: a sociological view. In W. Tseng and D. Y. H. Wu (eds) *Chinese culture and mental health* (pp. 29–46). London: Academic Press.

Kirmayer, L. J. 2000. Broken narratives: clinical encounters and the poetics of illness experience. In C. Mattingly and L. C. Garro (eds) *Narrative and the cultural construction of illness and healing* (pp. 153–180). Berkeley, US: University of California Press.

Kleinman, A. 1980. *Patients and healers in the context of culture: an exploration of the borderland between anthropology, medicine, and psychiatry.* Berkeley, CA, US: University of California Press.

Kleinman, A. 1982. Neurasthenia and depression: a study of somatization and culture in China. *Culture, Medicine and Psychiatry*, 6, 117–190.

Kleinman, A. 1988. *The illness narratives: suffering, healing, and the human condition.* New York: Basic Books.

Kleinman, A. 2010. Caregiving: its role in medicine and society in America and China. *Ageing International*, 35, 96–108.

Kleinman, A. and Kleinman, J. 1985. Somatization: the interconnections in Chinese society among culture, depressive experiences, and the meanings of pain. In A. Kleinman and B. Good (eds) *Culture and depression: studies in the anthropology and cross-cultural psychiatry of affect and disorder* (pp. 429–490). Berkeley, CA, US: University of California Press.

Kleinman, A., Eisenberg, L. and Good, B. 2006. Culture, illness, and care: clinical lessons from anthropologic and cross-cultural research. *Focus: the Journal of Lifelong Learning in Psychiatry*, 4 (1), 140–149.

Kleinman, A., Yan, Y., Jun, J., Lee, S., Zhang, E., Pan, T., Wu, F. and Guo, J. 2011. *Deep China: the moral life of the person: what anthropology and psychiatry tell us about China today.* Berkeley, US: University of California Press.

Knight, D. S. 2006. Madness and disability in contemporary Chinese film. *Journal of Medical Humanities*, 27, 93–103.

Kohrman, M. 2005. *Bodies of difference: experiences of disability and institutional advocacy in the making of modern China.* Berkeley, US: University of California Press.

Kong, S. 2008. Family matters: reconstructing the family on the Chinese television screen. In Y. Zhu, M. Keane and R. Bai (eds) *TV drama in China* (pp. 75–88). Hong Kong: Hong Kong University Press.

Korabik, K. 1993. Managerial women in the People's Republic of China: the Long March continues. *International Studies of Management and Organization*, 23 (4), 47–64.

Kung, W. W. 2001. Consideration of cultural factors in working with Chinese American families with a mentally ill patient. *Journal of Contemporary Human Services*, 82 (1), 97–107.

Labov, W. and Waletzky, J. 1997. Narrative analysis: oral versions of personal experience. *Journal of Narrative and Life History*, 7 (1–4), 3–38.

Lafrance, M. 2007. A bitter pill: a discursive analysis of women's medicalized accounts of depression. *Journal of Health Psychology*, 12 (1), 127–140.

Lai, D. W. L. 2007. Cultural predictors of caregiving burden of Chinese-Canadian family caregivers. *Canadian Journal on Aging*, 26 (S1), 133–148.

Lai, D. W. L. 2010. Filial piety, caregiving appraisal, and caregiving burden. *Research on Aging*, 32 (2), 200–223.

Lai, D. W. L. and Surood, S. 2009. Chinese health beliefs of older Chinese in Canada. *Journal of Aging and Health*, 21 (1), 38–62.

Laidlaw, K., Wang, D. H., Coelho, C. and Power, M. 2010. Attitudes to ageing and expectations for filial piety across Chinese and British cultures: a pilot exploratory evaluation. *Aging and Mental Health*, 14 (3), 283–292.

Lam, M. M. L., Pearson, V., Ng, R. M. K., Chiu, C. P.Y., Law, C. W. and Chen, E. Y. H. 2011. What does recovery from psychosis mean? Perceptions of young first-episode patients. *International Journal of Social Psychiatry*, 57 (6), 580–587.

Lam, R. C. 2006. Contradictions between traditional Chinese values and the actual performance: a study of the caregiving roles of the modern sandwich generation in Hong Kong. *Journal of Comparative Family Studies*, 37 (2), 299–313.

Lan, F. 2011. From the de-based literati to the de-based intellectual: a Chinese hypochondriac in Japan. *Modern Chinese Literature and Culture*, 23, 105–132.

Lee, D. T. S., Kleinman, J. and Kleinman, A. 2007. Rethinking depression: an ethnographic study of the experiences of depression among Chinese. *Harvard Review of Psychiatry*, 15 (1), 1–8.

Lee, H. K. [李洪根]. 2005. 似曾相識. 香港: 環球(國際)出版有限公司.

Lee, S. and Kleinman, A. 2007. Are somatoform disorders changing with time? The case of neurasthenia in China. *Psychosomatic Medicine*, 69, 846–849.

Lee, S., Chiu, M. Y. L., Tsang, A., Chui. H. and Kleinman, A. 2006. Stigmatizing experience and structural discrimination associated with the treatment of schizophrenia in Hong Kong. *Social Science and Medicine*, 62, 1685–1696.

Lefley, H. P. 1996. *Family caregiving in mental illness*. Thousand Oaks, CA, US: Sage.

Leung, J. C. B. 2001. Family support and community-based services in China. In I. Chi, N. L. Chappell and J. Lubben (eds) *Elderly Chinese in Pacific rim countries: social support and integration* (pp. 171–188). Hong Kong: Hong Kong University Press.

Leung, L. and Gallagher-Thompson, D. 2005. Stress management with a Chinese female caregiver in a family system. *Clinical Gerontologist*, 28 (3), 87–89.

Li, S. and Phillips, M. R. 1990. Witch doctors and mental illness in mainland China: a preliminary study. *The American Journal of Psychiatry*, 147 (2), 221–224.

Li, Y. and Lemke, D. 2004. A comparison study between American and Chinese societies: home caring for elders with Alzheimer's and memory impairments. *The Social Science Journal*, 41, 485–492.

Lieblich, A., Tuval-Mashiach, R. and Zilber, T. 1998. *Narrative research: reading, analysis and interpretation*. Thousand Oaks, CA, US: Sage.

Lin, K. 1981. Traditional Chinese medical beliefs and their relevance for mental illness and psychiatry. In A. Kleinman and T. Lin (eds) *Normal and abnormal behaviour in Chinese culture* (pp. 95–114). Dordrecht, The Netherlands: D. Reidel.

Lin, P. C. and Lu, C. M. 2005. Hip fracture: family caregivers' burden and related factors for older people in Taiwan. *Journal of Clinical Nursing*, 14, 719–726.

Lin, T., Tseng, W. and Yeh, E. 1995. Chinese culture, orientation, and coping. In T. Lin, W. Tseng and E. Yeh (eds) *Chinese society and mental health* (pp. 1–2). Hong Kong: Oxford University Press.

Linder, B. 2011. Trauma and truth: representations of madness in Chinese literature. *Journal of Medical Humanities*, 32, 291–303.

Link, B. and Phelan, J. 2001. Conceptualizing stigma. *Annual Review of Sociology*, 27, 363–385.

Link, B., Yang, L., Phelan, J. and Collins, P. 2004. Measuring mental illness stigma. *Schizophrenia Bulletin*, 30 (3), 511–541.

Liu, D., Hinton, L., Tran, C., Hinton, D. and Barker, J. C. 2008. Reexamining the relationships among dementia, stigma, and aging in immigrant Chinese and Vietnamese family caregivers. *Journal of Cross-Cultural Gerontology*, 23, 283–299.

Liu, W., Wang, P. C., Gray, H., Tang, P. C. Y., Kwo, E., Thompson, L. and Gallagher-Thompson, D. 2008. Client satisfaction with a stress reduction program for Chinese dementia caregivers. *Hallym International Journal of Aging*, 10 (2), 91–110.

Loo, C., Tong, B. and True, R. 1989. A bitter bean: mental health status and attitudes in Chinatown. *Journal of Community Psychology*, 17, 283–295.

Lothe, J. 2000. *Narrative in fiction and film: an introduction*. Oxford, UK: Oxford University Press.

Lupton, D. 2003. *Medicine as culture: illness, disease and the body in Western societies*. Thousand Oaks, CA, US: Sage.

Lysaker, P. H., Ringer, J., Maxwell, C., McGuire, A. and Lecomte, T. 2010. Personal narratives and recovery from schizophrenia. *Schizophrenia Research*, 121, 271–276.

McCabe, R. and Priebe, S. 2004. Explanatory models of illness in schizophrenia: comparison of four ethnic groups. *British Journal of Psychiatry*, 185, 25–30.

McDougall, B. and Louie, K. 1997. *The literature of China in the twentieth century*. London: Hurst & Co.

McKay, S. and Bonner, F. 2002. Evaluating illness in women's magazines. *Journal of Language and Social Psychology*, 21 (1), 53–67.

MacKenzie, A. E. and Holroyd, E. 1996. An exploration of the carers' perceptions of caregiving and caring responsibilities in Chinese families. *International Journal of Nursing Studies*, 33 (1), 1–12.

Mann, S. 2011. *Gender and sexuality in modern Chinese history*. New York: Cambridge University Press.

Metzger, T. A. 1981. Selfhood and authority in Neo-Confucian political culture. In A. Kleinman and T. Lin (eds) *Normal and abnormal behaviour in Chinese culture* (pp. 7–28). Dordrecht, The Netherlands: D. Reidel.

Miller, M. Z., Martin, P. G. and Beatty, K. C. 2005. Wholeness in a breaking world: narratives as sustenance for peace. In L. M. Harter, P. M. Japp and C. S. Beck (eds) *Narratives, health, and healing: communication theory, research, and practice* (pp. 295–316). Mahwah, NJ, US: L. Erlbaum Associates.

Milliken, P. J. 2001. Disenfranchised mothers: caring for an adult child with schizophrenia. *Health Care for Women International*, 22, 149–166.

Mishler, E. G. 1984. *The discourse of medicine: dialectics of medical interviews*. Norwood, NJ, US: Ablex.

Mishler, E. G. 1995. Models of narrative analysis. *Journal of Narrative and Life History*, 5 (2), 87–123.

Ng, R. M. K., Pearson, V. and Chen, E. Y. H. 2008a. What does recovery from schizophrenia mean? Perceptions of psychiatrists. *International Journal of Culture and Mental Health*, 1 (1), 73–84.

Ng, R. M. K., Pearson, V., Lam, M., Law, C. W., Chiu, C. P. Y. and Chen, E. Y. H. 2008b. What does recovery from schizophrenia mean? Perceptions of long-term patients. *International Journal of Social Psychiatry*, 54 (2), 118–130.

Ng, R. M. K., Pearson, V., Chen, E. E. Y. and Law, C. W. 2011. What does recovery from schizophrenia mean? Perceptions of medical students and trainee psychiatrists. *International Journal of Social Psychiatry*, 57 (3), 248–262.

Ng, R. M. K., Pearson, V., Pang, Y. W., Wong, N. S., Wong, N. C. and Chan F. M. 2012. The uncut jade: differing views of the potential of expert users on staff training and rehabilitation programmes for service users in Hong Kong. *International Journal of Social Psychiatry*, published online before print 4 January 2012, DOI: 10.1177/0020764011431540.

O'Brien, M. R. and Clark, D. 2010. Use of unsolicited first-person written illness narratives in research: systematic review. *Journal of Advanced Nursing*, 66 (8), 1671–1682.

Öhman, M. and Söderberg, S. 2004. The experiences of close relatives living with a person with serious chronic illness. *Qualitative Health Research*, 14 (3), 396–410.

O'Shaughnessy, M. and Stadler, J. 2008. *Media and society*. South Melbourne, Victoria, Australia: Oxford University Press.

Pearson, V. 1995a. *Mental health care in China: state policies, professional services and family responsibilities*. London: Gaskell.

Pearson, V. 1995b. Population policy and eugenics in China. *The British Journal of Psychiatry*, 167, 1–4.

Pearson, V. 1995c. Goods on which one loses: women and mental health in China. *Social Science and Medicine*, 41 (8), 1159–1173.

Pearson, V. 1996. The Chinese equation in mental health policy and practice. *International Journal of Law and Psychiatry*, 19 (3/4), 437–458.

Pearson, V. and Lam, P. 2002. On their own: caregivers in Guangzhou, China. In H. Lefley and D. Johnson (eds) *Family interventions in mental illness: international perspectives* (pp. 171–183). Westport, CT, US: Praeger.

Pearson, V. and Ning, S. P. 1997. Family care in schizophrenia: an undervalued resource. In N. Rhind and C. Chan (eds) *Social work intervention in health care: the Hong Kong scene* (pp. 317–337). Hong Kong: Hong Kong University Press.

Pearson, V. and Phillips, M. R. 1994. The social context of psychiatric rehabilitation in China. *British Journal of Psychiatry*, 165 (S24), 11–18.

Pearson, V. and Tsang, H. 2004. Duty, burden, and ambivalence: families of forensic psychiatric patients in Hong Kong. *International Journal of Law and Psychiatry*, 27, 361–374.

Pejlert, A. 2001. Being a parent of an adult son or daughter with severe mental illness receiving professional care: parents' narratives. *Health and Social Care in the Community*, 9 (4), 194–204.

Petrus, N. G. and Wing-chung, H. O. 2005. Experience in coping with Alzheimer's disease at home: a study of Chinese family caregivers. *Journal of Social Work in Disability and Rehabilitation*, 4 (4), 1–14.

Phillips, M. 1993. Strategies used by Chinese families coping with schizophrenia. In D. Davis and S. Harrell (eds) *Chinese families in the post-Mao era* (pp. 277–306). Berkeley, US: University of California Press.

Phillips, M., Pearson, V., Li, F. F., Xu, M. J. and Yang, L. 2002. Stigma and expressed emotion: a study of people with schizophrenia and their family members in China. *British Journal of Psychiatry*, 181, 488–493.

Pierret, J. 2003. The illness experience: state of knowledge and perspectives for research. *Sociology of Health and Illness*, 25, 4–22.

Pinnegar, S. and Daynes, J. G. 2007. Locating narrative inquiry historically: thematics in the turn to narrative. In D. J. Clandinin (ed.) *Handbook of narrative inquiry: mapping a methodology* (pp. 3–34). Thousand Oaks, CA, US: Sage.

Polanyi, L. 1989. *Telling the American story: a structural and cultural analysis of conversational storytelling.* Cambridge, MA, US: MIT Press.

Qiu, J. 2007. Ticking time bomb faced by China's ageing population. *The Lancet Neurology*, 6, 582–583.

Ramsay, G. 1997. *Beijing Review newstext: a comparative cross-cultural analysis of lexico-semantic and discourse structural features.* Unpublished doctoral dissertation. St. Lucia, QLD, Australia: The University of Queensland.

Ramsay, G. 2008. *Shaping minds: a discourse analysis of Chinese-language community mental health literature.* Amsterdam: John Benjamins.

Ramsay, G. 2010. Mainland Chinese family caregiver narratives in mental illness: disruption and continuity. *Asian Studies Review*, 34 (1), 83–103.

Ran, M. S., Xiang, M. Z., Chan, C. L. W., Leff, J., Simpson, P., Huang, M. S., Shan, Y. H. and Li, S. G. 2003. Effectiveness of psychoeducational intervention for rural Chinese families experiencing schizophrenia: a randomised control trial. *Social Psychiatry and Psychiatric Epidemiology*, 38, 69–75.

Ran, M. S., Xiang, M. Z., Simpson, P. and Chan, C. L. W. 2005. *Family-based mental health care in rural China.* Hong Kong: Hong Kong University Press.

Ricoeur, P. 1984. *Time and narrative.* Chicago, US: University of Chicago Press.

Riessman, C. K. 1993. *Narrative analysis.* Newbury Park, CA, US: Sage.

Riessman, C. K. 2000. 'Even if we don't have children [we] can live': stigma and infertility in south India. In C. Mattingly and L. C. Garro (eds) *Narrative and the cultural construction of illness and healing* (pp. 128–152). Berkeley, US: University of California Press.

Riessman, C. K. 2004. A thrice-told tale: new readings of an old story. In B. Hurwitz, T. Greenhalgh and V. Skultans (eds) *Narrative research in health and illness* (pp. 309–324). Malden, MA, US: BMJ Books.

Roberts, R. A. 2010. *Maoist model theatre: the semiotics of gender and sexuality in the Chinese Cultural Revolution (1966–1976).* Leiden, The Netherlands: Brill.

Rojas, C. 2011. Of canons and cannibalism: a psycho-immunological reading of 'Diary of a Madman.' *Modern Chinese Literature and Culture*, 23, 47–76.

Roy, W. 2009. The word is colander: language loss and narrative voice in fictional Canadian Alzheimer's narratives. *Canadian Literature*, 203, 41–63.

Scambler, G. 2004. Re-framing stigma: felt and enacted stigma and challenges to the sociology of chronic and disabling conditions. *Social Theory and Health*, 2, 29–46.

Shapiro, J. 2011. Illness narratives: reliability, authenticity and the empathic witness. *Medical Humanities*, 37 (2), 68–72.

Skultans, V. 2003. From damaged nerves to masked depression: inevitability and hope in Latvian psychiatric narratives. *Social Science and Medicine*, 56, 2421–2431.

Song, Y. and Wang, J. 2010. Overview of Chinese research on senile dementia in mainland China. *Ageing Research Reviews*, 9S, S6–S12.

Sontag, S. 1989. *Illness as metaphor and AIDS and its metaphors.* New York: Picador.

Squire, C. 2005. Reading narratives. *Group Analysis*, 38 (1), 91–107.

Squire, C. 2007. *HIV in South Africa: talking about the big thing*. Hoboken, US: Taylor & Francis.

Stein, C., Mann, L. and Hunt, M. 2007. Ever onward: the personal strivings of young adults coping with serious mental illness and the hopes of their parents. *American Journal of Orthopsychiatry*, 77 (1), 104–112.

Stern, S., Doolan, M., Staples, E., Szmukler, G.L. and Eisler, I. 1999. Disruption and reconstruction: narrative insights into the experience of family members caring for a relative diagnosed with serious mental illness. *Family Process*, 38 (3), 353–369.

Stewart, A. J. and Malley, J. E. 2004. Women of 'The Greatest Generation': feeling on the margin of social history. In C. Daiute and C. Lightfoot (eds) *Narrative analysis: studying the development of individuals in society* (pp. 223–244). Thousand Oaks, CA, US: Sage.

Stoltz, P., Willman, A. and Udén, G. 2006. The meaning of support as narrated by family carers who care for a senior relative at home. *Qualitative Health Research*, 16 (5), 594–610.

Tebbe, J. 2008. Landscapes of remembrance: home and memory in the nineteenth-century Bürgertum. *Journal of Family History*, 33 (2), 195–215.

Thomas, C. 2010. Negotiating the contested terrain of narrative methods in illness contexts. *Sociology of Health and Illness*, 32 (4), 647–660.

Thornborrow, J. and Coates, J. 2005. The sociolinguistics of narrative: identity, performance, culture. In J. Thornborrow and J. Coates (eds) *The sociolinguistics of narrative* (pp. 1–16). Amsterdam: John Benjamins.

Ting-Toomey, S. 1999. *Communicating across cultures*. New York: Guilford Press.

Toolan, M. 2001. *Narrative: a critical linguistic introduction*. New York: Routledge.

Traphagan, J. 2000. *Taming oblivion: aging bodies and the fear of senility in Japan*. New York: State University of New York Press.

Trevaskes, S. 2007. *Courts and criminal justice in contemporary China*. Lanham, US: Lexington.

Tseng, W. 1986. Chinese psychiatry: development and characteristics. In J. L. Cox (ed.) *Transcultural psychiatry* (pp. 274–290). London: Crown Helm.

Tuck, I., du Mont, P., Evans, G. and Shupe, J. 1997. The experience of caring for an adult child with schizophrenia. *Archives of Psychiatric Nursing*, XI (3), 118–125.

Vanderstaay, L. M. C. 2011. *A textual analysis of female consciousness in twenty-first century Chinese women directors' films*. Unpublished doctoral dissertation. St Lucia, QLD, Australia: The University of Queensland.

Wang, P. C., Tong, H. Q., Liu, W., Long, S., Leung, L. Y. L., Yau, E. and Gallagher-Thompson, D. 2006. Working with Chinese American families. In G. Yeo and D. Gallagher-Thompson (eds) *Ethnicity and the dementias* (pp. 173–188). New York: Routledge.

Wedding, D., Boyd, M. A. and Niemiec, R. M. 2005. *Movies and mental illness: using films to understand psychopathology*. Toronto, Canada: Hogrefe & Huber.

Williams, B. and Healy, D. 2001. Perceptions of illness causation among new referrals to a community mental health team: 'explanatory model' or 'exploratory map'? *Social Science and Medicine*, 53, 465–476.

Wiltshire, J. 2000. Biography, pathography, and the recovery of meaning. *Cambridge Quarterly*, 29 (4), 409–422.

Wisdom, J. P., Bruce, K., Saedi, G. A., Weis, T. and Green, C. A. 2008. 'Stealing me from myself': identity and recovery in personal accounts of mental illness. *Australian and New Zealand Journal of Psychiatry*, 42, 489–495.

Wong, D. 2000. Stress factors and mental health of carers with relatives suffering from schizophrenia in Hong Kong: implications for culturally sensitive practices. *British Journal of Social Work*, 30, 365–382.

Wong, D., Tsui, H., Pearson, V., Chen, E. and Chiu, S. N. 2003. Changing health beliefs on causations of mental illness and their impacts on family burdens and the mental health of Chinese caregivers in Hong Kong. *International Journal of Mental Health*, 32 (2), 84–98.

Wong, D., Tsui, H., Pearson, V., Chen, E. and Chiu, S. N. 2004. Family burdens, Chinese health beliefs, and the mental health of Chinese caregivers in Hong Kong. *Transcultural Psychiatry*, 41 (4), 497–513.

Woods, A. 2011. The limits of narrative: provocations for the medical humanities. *Medical Humanities*, 37 (2), 73–78.

Wu, E., Rapport, F., Jones, K. and Greenhalgh, T. 2004. Soldiers become casualties: doctors' accounts of the SARS epidemic. In B. Hurwitz, T. Greenhalgh and V. Skultans (eds) *Narrative research in health and illness* (pp. 37–51). Malden, MA, US: BMJ Books.

Xiang, M., Ran, M. and Li, S. 1994. A controlled evaluation of psychoeducational family intervention in a rural Chinese community. *British Journal of Psychiatry*, 165, 544–548.

Xiong, W., Phillips, M. R., Hu, X., Wang, R., Dai, Q., Kleinman, J. and Kleinman, A. 1994. Family-based intervention for schizophrenic patients in China: a randomised controlled trial. *British Journal of Psychiatry*, 165, 239–247.

Xu, J. H. 2008. Family saga serial dramas and reinterpretation of cultural traditions. In Y. Zhu, M. Keane and R. Bai (eds) *TV drama in China* (pp. 33–46). Hong Kong: Hong Kong University Press.

Yamashita, M. and Forsyth, D. 1998. Family coping with mental illness: an aggregate from two studies, Canada and United States. *Journal of the American Psychiatric Nurses Association*. 4, 1–8.

Yang, L. H. 2007. Application of mental illness stigma theory to Chinese societies: synthesis and new directions. *Singapore Medical Journal*, 48 (11), 977–985.

Yang, L. H. and Kleinman, A. 2008. 'Face' and the embodiment of stigma in China: the cases of schizophrenia and AIDS. *Social Science and Medicine*, 67, 398–408.

Yang, L. H. and Pearson, V. J. 2002. Understanding families in their own context: schizophrenia and structural family therapy in Beijing. *Journal of Family Therapy*, 24, 233–257.

Yang, X. 2011. Configuring female sickness and recovery: Chen Ran and Anni Baobei. *Modern Chinese Literature and Culture*, 23, 169–196.

Yao, G. [姚贵忠] (ed.). 2000. 精神疾病康复文集. 北京: 中国科学技术出版社.

Yao, G. [姚贵忠] (ed.). 2007. 我的世界从此改变 —《精神康复报》十年精粹. n.p.

Yip, K. S. 2005. Family intervention and services for persons with mental illness in the People's Republic of China. *Journal of Family Social Work*, 9 (1), 65–82.

Yip, K. S. 2007. *Mental health service in the People's Republic of China: current status and future developments*. New York: Nova Science Publishers.

Yu, S. W. K. and Chau, R. C. M. 1997. The sexual division of care in mainland China and Hong Kong. *International Journal of Urban and Regional Research*, 21 (4), 607–619.

Zhan, H. J. 2006. Joy and sorrow: explaining Chinese caregivers' reward and stress. *Journal of Aging Studies*, 20, 27–38.

Zhang, M., Yan, H., Yao, C., Ye, J., Yu, Q., Chen, P., Guo, L., Yang, J., Qu, G., Wong, Z., Cai, J., Shen, M., Hou, J., Wang, L., Zhang, Y., Zhang, B., Orley, J. and Gittelman, M.

1993. Effectiveness of psychoeducation of relatives of schizophrenic patients: a prospective cohort study in five cities of China. *International Journal of Mental Health*, 22 (1), 47–59.

Zhang, M., Wang, M., Li, J. and Phillips, M. 1994. Randomised-control trial of family intervention for 78 first-episode male schizophrenic patients: an 18-month study in Suzhou, Jiangsu. *British Journal of Psychiatry*, 165 (S24), 96–102.

Zhu, Y., Keane, M. and Bai, R. 2008. Introduction. In Y. Zhu, M. Keane and R. Bai (eds) *TV drama in China* (pp. 1–18). Hong Kong: Hong Kong University Press.

Index

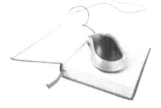
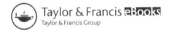

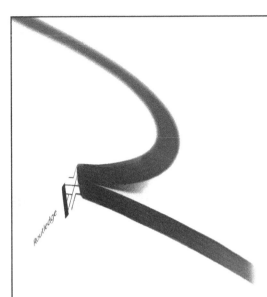
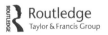

ROUTLEDGE Revivals

Are there some elusive titles you've been searching for but thought you'd never be able to find?

Well this may be the end of your quest. We now offer a fantastic opportunity to discover past brilliance and purchase previously out of print and unavailable titles by some of the greatest academic scholars of the last 120 years.

Routledge Revivals is an exciting new programme whereby key titles from the distinguished and extensive backlists of the many acclaimed imprints associated with Routledge are re-issued.

The programme draws upon the backlists of Kegan Paul, Trench & Trubner, Routledge & Kegan Paul, Methuen, Allen & Unwin and Routledge itself.

Routledge Revivals spans the whole of the Humanities and Social Sciences, and includes works by scholars such as Emile Durkheim, Max Weber, Simone Weil and Martin Buber.

FOR MORE INFORMATION

Please email us at **reference@routledge.com** or visit:
www.routledge.com/books/series/Routledge_Revivals

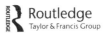

Milton Keynes UK
Ingram Content Group UK Ltd.
UKHW040052071024
449327UK00019B/496